Idol Worship in Chinese Society

T0187873

This book introduces psychosocial studies of idol worship in Chinese societies. It reviews how idol worship is perceived in Chinese culture, history, and philosophy as well as how it differs from the concept of celebrity worship that is more dominant in Western literature. Using a pioneering hexagonal model of idol worship, this book explains how idol worship is affected by various demographic and dispositional variables as well as the cognitive and social functions of idols and idol worship. Finally, it discusses idol worship from a contemporary Chinese perspective, including emotional, interpersonal, and social learning aspects, and ends with a discussion of the moral development perspective.

Xiaodong Yue 岳曉東 is assistant dean, School of Graduate Studies, College of Liberal Arts and Social Sciences, and associate professor, Department of Social and Behavioral Sciences at City University of Hong Kong. He earned his BA degree in English language and literature at Beijing Second Foreign Languages Institute in 1982, his MA degree in education from Tufts University in 1987, and his EdD degree in psychology from Harvard University in 1993. He has taught psychology courses at the Department of Educational Psychology of Chinese University of Hong Kong (1993–1996) and at the Department of Applied Social Sciences of City University of Hong Kong (since 1997). He has published widely on issues of creativity, humor, resilience, and adolescent idol worship in Chinese society. He is an adjunct professor of over 20 universities in China as well as an ad hoc reviewer of ten international journals of psychology and education around the world. He is also the founding chair of the Division of Counseling Psychology of the Hong Kong Psychological Society. He has been invited to give keynote addresses at various conferences in China and around the world. (Contact him at ssxdyue@cityu.edu.hk.)

Chau-kiu Cheung is associate professor, Department of Social and Behavioral Sciences at City University of Hong Kong. He has recently published on the topics of emerging adulthood, child abuse, resilience, character education, moral development, peer influence, and class mobility. His current research addresses issues of idolatry, violence, distress, career, and prosociality. (Contact him at ssjacky@cityu.edu.hk.)

Routledge Studies in Asian Behavioural Sciences

Series Editor: T. Wing Lo

City University of Hong Kong

Archaeology of Psychotherapy in Korea
A Study of Korean Therapeutic Work and Professional Growth
Haeyoung Jeong

Hidden Youth and the Virtual World
The Process of Social Censure and Empowerment
Gloria Hongyee Chan

Psychoanalysis in Hong Kong
The Absent, the Present, and the Reinvented
Diego Busiol

Psycho-Criminological Perspective of Criminal Justice in Asia
Research and Practices in Hong Kong, Singapore, and Beyond
Edited by Heng Choon (Oliver) Chan and Samuel M.Y. Ho

Humour and Chinese Culture
A Psychological Perspective
Yue Xiao Dong

Idol Worship in Chinese Society
A Psychological Approach
Xiaodong Yue and Chau-kiu Cheung

For the full list of titles in the series visit: https://www.routledge.com/Routledge-Studies-in-Asian-Behavioural-Sciences/book-series/RABS

Idol Worship in Chinese Society

A Psychological Approach

Xiaodong Yue and Chau-kiu Cheung

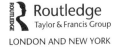

Routledge
Taylor & Francis Group

LONDON AND NEW YORK

First published 2019
by Routledge
2 Park Square, Milton Park, Abingdon, Oxon OX14 4RN

and by Routledge
52 Vanderbilt Avenue, New York, NY 10017, USA

First issued in paperback 2020

*Routledge is an imprint of the Taylor & Francis Group, an informa
business*

British Library Cataloguing in Publication Data
A catalogue record for this book is available from the British Library

Library of Congress Cataloging in Publication Data
Names: Yue, Xiaodong, 1959- author. | Cheung, Chau-kiu, author.
Title: Idol worship in Chinese society : a psychological approach /
Xiaodong Yue and Chau-kiu Cheung.
Description: First Edition. | New York : Routledge, 2019. |
Series: Routledge studies in asian behavioural sciences | Includes
bibliographical references and index.
Identifiers: LCCN 2018026478 | ISBN 9780415788861 (hardback) |
ISBN 9781315223124 (e-book)
Subjects: LCSH: Idols and images—China—Worship. |
Psychology—China.
Classification: LCC BL485 .Y84 2019 | DDC 299.5/11218—dc23
LC record available at https://lccn.loc.gov/2018026478

ISBN 13: 978-0-367-58421-4 (pbk)
ISBN 13: 978-0-415-78886-1 (hbk)

Typeset in ITC Galliard Std
by Cenveo® Publisher Services

Contents

Preface

This book is the realization of the two coauthors' dream as well as an attempt to combine our specialized knowledge in two interrelated disciplines: psychology for Xiaodong Yue and sociology for Chau-kiu Cheung. For more than two decades, we conducted programmatic studies examining adolescent idolatrous behaviors in many Chinese cities, including Beijing, Changsha, Guangzhou, Hangzhou, Hong Kong, Nanjing, and Shenzhen. Over time, we have found ourselves to be the pioneering scholars of idol worship studies in Chinese society, and our works have been helpful to researchers all over the world. For this reason, we have talked for years about coauthoring a book to summarize our empirical findings and theoretical propositions. Now, we have the book!

We are sincerely grateful for Routledge Press for making this project possible. We are particularly grateful to Ms. ShengBin Tang for her kind guidance and patience and for allowing us to write this book in the best possible way. We are also very grateful to Professor Tit-Wing Lo, our dear colleague at CityU, for motivating us to contribute a volume to the book series on Chinese social behaviors of which he is the editor. Meanwhile, we are very grateful to Ms. Neelam A. Hiranandani for helping to write, edit, and proofread chapters in this book.

We believe this book will inform you of the critical concepts, constructs, and theories about adolescent idolatrous behaviors in Chinese societies, particularly in Hong Kong. We also hope this book will encourage you to think critically about empirical studies and theoretical propositions about idol worship studies conducted in Chinese society. Even with its present scope, we realize that many topics and themes in idol worship are not covered in this book; we hope this book will inspire others to pursue these topics later. Alternatively, as we often say in Chinese, we want to attract jade by laying bricks (抛磚引玉), which means offering crude remarks to draw forth better ones.

Above all, we hope this work will contribute to cross-cultural understanding of idol worship around the world, as it is becoming increasingly prevalent in all corners of the globe. We also firmly believe that idol worship, during adolescence in particular, can exert positive influences on worshippers' mentality and psychosocial development as long as they can demystify the glamorous and magnificent aspects of their admired idols and identify with their socially desirable dispositions or traits. This is the theme of this book.

Finally, we thank all those who read this book and look forward to discussing the themes with you.

Xiaodong Yue
Chau-kiu Cheung

1 Idol worship and related concepts

Idols, celebrities, and idol figures

The *Merriam-Webster Dictionary* defines *idol* (偶像) as a representation or symbol of an object of worship. Broadly, idols are false gods, enchanting figures inducing love and admiration for their perceived power and grandeur (Engle and Kasser 2005).

Idols include diverse contemporary, historic, and fictional figures. Historically and prehistorically, idols have been religious, ritualistic figures worshipped as protectors of personal health, wealth, and all things valuable. Today, the meaning of *idol* has been extended from the broad historical category to include admired luminaries, recreational stars, and political leaders, beyond social, political, or religious backgrounds. Typically, idol worshippers perceive their idols as being physically attractive, greatly talented, highly achieving, or having high status.

Idols may be religious idols, such as Jesus Christ, Buddha, and Allah; ethnic idols, such as gods and goddesses of land, heaven, and rain; sage/luminary idols, such as scientific and philosophical figures; and recreational idols, such as pop, movie, and sports stars (Yue and Liang 2009). The meanings of *idol* and *celebrity* overlap. Idols are not always celebrities, but they must be distinctive and are likely to be revered for a long time. Celebrities, on the other hand, are entities accorded shorter-term fame and public attention through the mass media. Celebrity status is often associated with wealth and fame.

An *idol figure* (偶像人物) is typically a celebrity, hero, or luminary (Maltby et al. 2004). In Hong Kong, idol figures are usually "tri-star people" (三星人物)—that is, generally young, attractive, glamorous, wealthy, and energetic pop stars (歌星), movie stars (影星), and sports stars (体坛明星) (Yue and Cheung 2000). In contrast, luminaries may appear humble and ordinary but have achieved distinction in fields such as business, education, politics, and sciences (Cheung and Yue 2002, 2003a, 2003b; Yue and Cheung 2000). Hong Kong's mass media and the commercialization of the entertainment industry has encouraged the worship of pop idols (Cheung and Yue 2000; Leung 1999; Yue and Cheung 2000a, 2000b, 2000; Yue et al. 2000). Similar patterns of idol selection and idol worship are found in nearby regions, such as China, Japan, Malaysia, Singapore, and South Korea (e.g., Swami et al. 2011).

What does *idol* mean in the Chinese language?

In Chinese classics, the word *idol* means a Dogū doll, either a wooden puppet or a clay statue. In the early second-century Chinese dictionary *Shuowen* (《說文》), *ou* (偶 *kirito*) means a wooden person (偶，桐人也). The first reference to idols comes from the *Historical Records of Yin Ji* (《史記·殷本紀》), which states that in the late Shang dynasty (1600–1046 BCE), Emperor Wu Yi made a wooden figure representing God to fight with him. Wu Yi won the fight and assumed that God was merely a useless figure deserving humiliation, so he covered the wooden figure with blood, hung it high, and shot at it, calling it the "heavenly shooting." After reigning for only four years, Wu Yi was hunting one day near the Yellow River and was fatally struck by lightning.

"殷商後期，帝武乙無道，為偶人，謂之天神，與之博，令人為行，天神不勝，乃繆辱之。為革囊盛血，仰而射之，命曰 '射天' 后猎于河渭之间。暴雷震死"

The moral is that if you offend God, you will be punished.

Fans and fandom

The *Merriam-Webster Dictionary* defines a *fan* (粉丝) as "either an enthusiastic devotee (as of a sport or a performing art) usually as a spectator or an ardent admirer or enthusiast (as of a celebrity or a pursuit) <science-fiction fans>." *Fandom* refers to the state or attitude of being a fan. The literature of leisure studies commonly uses the terms *serious leisure* (Cheng et al. 2017) and *serious sports fans* (Toffoletti 2017) to indicate that fandom (星迷) includes affectionate and committed admiration of and pursuit of celebrities (Stever 2013). *Serious fans* show their interest and commitment by writing letters to admired celebrities, attending fan gatherings, joining fan clubs, and holding extensive memorabilia collections (Stever 1994). Levels of fandom can be classified: fans who have the highest levels have an obsessive, pathological interest that interferes with normal life; fans who have normal levels are interested in celebrities for their ability to entertain; fans who have the lowest levels have little or no interest in celebrities (Stever 1994, 2009).

In a survey of 2,000 Hong Kong secondary school students, about 70% reported having at least one idol, mostly artists or stars (So and Chan 1992). They also reported being major fans of pop music and pop stars (Wong and Ma 1997), usually Chinese stars (Wan 1997). Adolescent girls were more likely than adolescent boys to join fan clubs (Cheng 1997).

Pop star idolization is also prevalent in Taiwan, with variations among idol categories and reasons for idolization (Lin and Lin 2007); that is, adolescents are most attracted to media stars. Furthermore, idolization was negatively correlated with idols' wealth and noncorrelated with idols' personality traits. In summary, young people in Hong Kong, Mainland China, and Taiwan tend to idolize tri-stars and admire role models.

Wei Jie—The idol who was killed by being watched

Wei Jie (衛玠)[1] is the only person in Chinese history who died of fatigue from being watched too much. The *Book of Jin Wei: Jie Biography* (《晋书·卫玠傳》) explains that he was so handsome (卫玠 是历史上唯一因为太帅了而被人"看"死的美男子。《晋书·卫玠传》："京师人士闻其姿容, 观者如堵 。玠劳疾遂甚, 永嘉六年卒, 时年二十七, 时人谓玠被看杀 。) that whenever he appeared in public, a wall of spectators surrounded him. He was so exhausted by the attention that he died at age 27. Later, people said the attention killed him.

《晋書·衛玠傳》："京師人士聞其姿容, 觀者如堵 。 玠勞疾遂甚, 永嘉六年卒, 時年二十七, 時人謂玠被看殺 。"

Idol worship, idolatry, and celebrity worship

The term *idol worship* (偶像崇拜) literally means worship of images or figures other than a Supreme Being for gaining power, protection, or fantasized intimacy. According to *Wikipedia*, the interchangeable term *idolatry* (偶像崇拜) refers to the worship of a physical image, such as a statue or icon. Similarly, the term *celebrity worship* (名人崇拜) focuses on pathologically motivated fan behaviors.

Idol worship indicates unilateral attachment to a figure. Such worship features frequent fantasies that exaggerate or idealize the idol's personal attributes (Fromm 1967; Yue and Cheung 2000a, 2000b). Idol worship is an imagined and nonreciprocal *parasocial* (人际互动) relationship (McCutcheon et al. 2002). As the world becomes increasingly globalized and modernized, the most likely idols are pop stars, celebrities, or sports heroes admired for their talents, achievements, status, and/or physical appearance (Adams-Price and Greene 1990; McCutcheon et al. 2003; Yue and Cheung 2000a, 2000b). They must be attractive to draw admiration from young people (Atkin and Block 1983).

Different kinds of idol worship

Idol worship and celebrity worship are measured in different ways (Cheung and Yue 2011; Maltby et al. 2004). Idol worship is a social phenomenon that forges false perceptions, intense attachments, and admiration of idol figures (Yue and Cheung 2000). Adolescents in Hong Kong tend to idolize media stars (明星偶像), whereas adolescents in Mainland China tend to worship both media stars and social luminaries (杰出人物偶像; Yue and Cheung 2000a, 2002).

More specifically, young people tend to worship the tri-stars (pop stars, movie stars, and sports stars), DJs, and fashion models for their glamour, wealth, carefree lifestyles, and unconventional behavior. Luminaries, in contrast, are typically outstanding scientists, politicians, writers, artists, and businesspeople admired for their personal achievements, social influence, dispositional charisma, and/or philosophies.

Idol worship includes three broad categories (Yue and Leung 2009): (1) *religious idol worship* (宗教型偶像崇拜) indicates religious ritualistic worship of revered figures, such as Jesus, Muhammad, and Buddha; religious worship originated from the worship of nature and perceptions of the Supreme Being (Yue 1999); (2) *ideological idol worship* (思想型偶像崇拜) indicates deep admiration for distinctive politicians, scientists, philosophers, and public figures who serve as role models for emulating ideal behaviors, verbalizations, expressions, personality characteristics, temperamental characteristics, personal conduct, and career achievements (Field 1981; Yue et al. 2003); and (3) *recreational idol worship* (娱乐型偶像崇拜) indicates adoration of music and movie stars for their talents, merits, status, or beauty (Yue and Cheung 2000b); it indicates unilateral attachment to idealized fantasy figures (Fromm 1967) showing, for example, trendy hairstyles, clothing, wealth, prestige, and lifestyles (Yue 1999).

Adolescent idol worship (青少年偶像崇拜), on the other hand, occurs when adolescents form a *secondary attachment* to a celebrity (Davidson 1983; Erikson 1968). That is, they have shifted their affectional attachment from nurturing parents to a more intimate, romantic attachment to fantasized distant celebrity figures (Erikson 1968; Freud 1922/1951; Greene and Adams-Price 1990).

On the positive side, attachments may allow adolescents to explore, experiment, and find stress relief. Before adolescents assume their permanent identity, they typically begin with exploration (Marcia 1980). By identifying with idols, they acquire ideals and values that will guide them in forming their adult roles (Erikson 1964, 1968). Although we know that idolization is important for identity formation, researchers have provided largely sporadic, unsystematic, and empirically tenuous studies showing that young people are most likely to nominate movie stars as their idols (Emanuel 1990) or to idolize pop musicians and singers and imagine themselves as musicians (Jeffrey 1991). They also admire individuals who have acquired significant income and prestige.

Differences between star idols and role models

As stated, media stars are idolized for being extraordinary, passionate, romantic, or irresistible. In contrast, role models are revered for being worthy, realistic, practical, and successful (Yue and Cheung 2000b). Idols and role models can be differentiated according to a hexagonal model comprising three pairs of contrasting concepts: *idealism* (理想化) versus *realism* (现实化), *romanticism* (浪漫化) versus *rationalism* (理性化), and *absolutism* (绝对化) versus *relativism* (相对化;

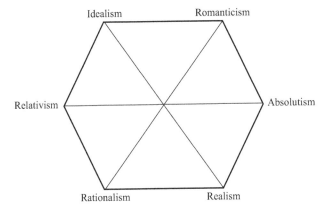

Figure 1.1 Hexagonal model for differentiating between idols and role models

Figure 1.1). Empirical support for the model was provided by an analysis of students in Nanjing and Hong Kong based on multidimensional scaling differentiation of the contrasting concepts (Figures 1.2 and 1.3; Yue and Cheung 2000a, 2000b).

The differentials were significant in ratings for romanticism, rationalism, idealism, and realism (Table 1.1). Gender was a significant source of variation in the differential rating for rationalism and realism. Place (Hong Kong vs. Nanjing) also contributed significant variation in rating differentials for absolutism.

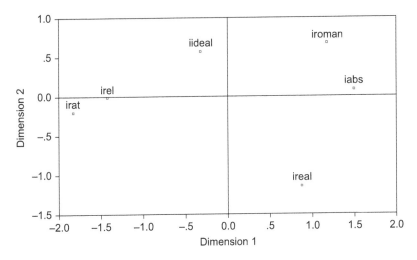

Figure 1.2 Configuration of idol worshipping derived from pooled Hong Kong and Nanjing data

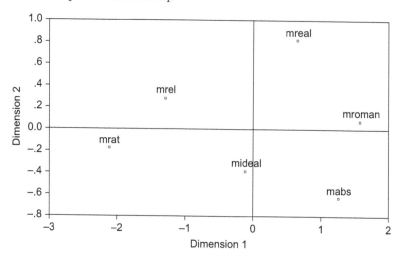

Figure 1.3 Configuration of role modeling derived from pooled Hong Kong and Nanjing
data

The three significant differences were clarified in the adjusted means. The relative importance of rationalism and realism as criteria for choosing role models rather than idols was more salient among girls (64.2 vs. 55.7) than boys (65.9 vs. 60.0). Concerning place effects on significant variations in the differential, students in Hong Kong were more focused on absolutism when choosing role models (38.6) rather than idols (34.6). Students in Nanjing emphasized absolutism slightly more when choosing idols (27.3) rather than role models (25.6).

Accordingly, students generally showed significant differentials in ratings for romanticism, rationalism, idealism, and realism in the expected direction (Table 1.1).

As expected, students placed more value on romanticism and idealism when they chose idols (m = 35.9 and 48.7; Table 1.2) rather than role models (m = 30.1 and 44.4). However, when they chose role models rather than

Table 1.1 F-values for testing differentials in ratings between idols
and role models from repeated-measures analysis of variance

Attributes	Overall	Place	Gender	Education
Romanticism	25.0*	1.6	0.9	1.1
Rationalism	54.8*	2.7	9.5*	0.0
Idealism	18.5*	1.9	0.0	2.0
Realism	31.2*	2.5	8.8*	3.4
Absolutism	0.3	4.9*	2.1	0.0
Relativism	0.8	2.5	0.1	0.1

Note
*p < .05 (two-tailed)

Table 1.2 Adjusted means estimated from repeated-measures analysis of variance

Attributes	Referent	Overall	Hong Kong	Nanjing	Boy	Girl	High school	University
Romanticism	Idol	35.9	34.9	33.6	36.3	32.3	40.4	28.1
Romanticism	Model	30.1	31.7	27.5	31.5	27.7	35.6	23.6
Rationalism	Idol	57.0	61.5	54.1	60.0	55.7	56.4	59.2
Rationalism	Model	63.7	70.0	60.1	65.9	64.2	62.4	67.7
Idealism	Idol	48.7	50.6	47.5	49.4	48.7	52.2	46.0
Idealism	Model	44.4	49.1	43.2	47.1	45.1	47.9	44.3
Realism	Idol	31.5	35.4	28.7	35.1	28.9	36.4	27.6
Realism	Model	35.1	39.2	32.2	37.1	34.3	40.8	30.6
Absolutism	Idol	30.1	34.6	27.3	35.0	26.9	35.2	26.7
Absolutism	Model	28.6	38.6	25.6	34.5	29.6	37.4	26.8
Relativism	Idol	55.1	58.0	53.1	55.8	55.3	56.9	54.2
Relativism	Model	56.6	55.8	55.7	57.0	54.6	55.9	55.6

idols, they placed more emphasis on rationalism and realism ($m = 57.0$ and 31.5). Although the differences were nonsignificant, absolutism was more important for choosing idols rather than role models ($m = 30.1$ vs. 28.6), and relativism was slightly more important for choosing role models rather than idols ($m = 56.6$ vs. 55.1).

The analysis also examined whether the differentials held for students of different education levels, genders, and locations. Results showed that background characteristics accounted for only three significant variations in the differentials. Both boys and girls indicated that rationalism and realism were more important for choosing role models rather than idols (adjusted $m = 60.0$, 55.7, 35.1, 28.9). Nanjing students felt that absolutism was more important for choosing idols than for choosing role models (adjusted $m = 27.3$ vs. 25.6), but Hong Kong students favored absolutism for choosing role models (adjusted $m = 38.6$ vs. 34.6).

In summary, for Chinese youth, idealism, romanticism, and absolutism were more important for selecting idols, whereas realism, rationalism, and relativism were more important for selecting role models. The differential selection pattern was more evident for young people in Hong Kong and Nanjing than in the other locations studied. Rationalism and relativism were significantly more important for choosing role models rather than idols, especially for girls. In comparison with university students, high school students regarded realism to be significantly more descriptive of role models. The findings imply the conceptual importance of distinguishing, as explicitly as possible, how idols differ from role models when we examine why young people admire significant people. Cherishing an idol rather than a role model could have quite different motivational implications and consequences. In fact, young people are likely to overly enhance or idealize the attributes of idol figures (e.g., Fromm 1967), but they are likely to admire role models when they perceive that they share some similarities with them (e.g., Schunk 1987).

Nomination studies of idol worship in Chinese societies

A pioneering study of adolescent idol worship examined 826 high school and university students: 167 high school students and 110 university students from Hong Kong, and 224 high school students and 325 university students from Nanjing (Cheung and Yue 2003a, 2004; Yue and Cheung 2000, 2002). Hong Kong participants were significantly more likely than participants in Nanjing to indicate more idealism-romanticism-absolutism (IRA) and significantly less realism-rationalism-relativism (RRR) toward celebrities (Table 1.3). Close to 75% of the favorite idols selected by Hong Kong university students and 86% of the favorite idols selected by Hong Kong high school students were IRA celebrities. In contrast, only 61% of the favorite idols selected by Nanjing high school students and 22% of the favorite idols selected by Nanjing university students were IRA celebrities. The most striking finding is that Hong Kong university students selected 3.5 times more IRA celebrities than did Nanjing university students. More than 96% of the role models selected by Hong Kong high school students and 91% of the role models selected by Nanjing high school students were RRR celebrities. In contrast, 82% of the favorite role models selected by Hong Kong university students and 61% of the favorite role models selected by Hong Kong high school students were RRR celebrities.

Intriguingly, nearly 18% of the role models selected by Hong Kong university students and 40% of the role models selected by Hong Kong high school students were IRA celebrities. Equally intriguing is that nearly 30% of the role models selected by Nanjing university students and nearly 20% of the role models selected by Nanjing high school students were public role models. This shows that public role models, however ordinary and common they may appear, still attract the admiration of young people. These findings support the assumption that young people in Hong Kong, in contrast with their counterparts in Nanjing, idolize IRA celebrities. It also supports the assumption that adolescent idol worship decreases with age (White and O'Brien 1999; Yue 1999).

Significant social differences in Hong Kong's and China's youth culture may explain the selection differences (Table 1.4). Hong Kong youth tend to be strongly driven by consumerist needs (Chan et al. 1998) and to be highly influenced by

Table 1.3 F-values for testing ratings for idols and role models from repeated-measures analysis of variance

Attributes	Place	Gender	Education	Order
Romanticism	4.4*	11.5*	36.2*	1.6
Rationalism	35.6*	0.9	0.2	9.1*
Idealism	10.6*	0.4	21.2*	0.1
Realism	12.0*	28.4*	47.3*	4.2*
Absolutism	30.0*	12.4*	41.8*	0.1
Relativism	6.1*	0.1	11.3*	0.7

Note
*$p < .05$ (two-tailed)

Table 1.4 Comparison of frequency counts for idols and role models selected by university and high school students in Hong Kong and Nanjing[a]

	Idols								Role models							
	University students				High school students				University students				High school students			
	Hong Kong (total = 163)[b]		Nanjing (total = 395)		Hong Kong (total = 316)		Nanjing (total = 306)		Hong Kong (total = 118)		Nanjing (total = 387)		Hong Kong (total = 165)		Nanjing (total = 341)	
Celebrities	No.	%	No.	%	No.	%	No.	%	No.	%	No.	%	No.	%	No.	%
A. Idealism-romanticism-absolutism oriented																
Singers[c]	72	44.2	38	9.6	187	59.2	67	21.9	9	7.6	1	0.3	29	17.6	11	3.2
Movie actors	30	18.4	25	6.3	54	17.1	47	15.4	8	6.8	4	1.0	20	12.1	4	1.2
Athletes	20	12.3	25	6.3	30	9.5	72	23.5	4	3.4	12	3.1	16	9.7	16	4.7
Total	122	74.8	88	22.3	271	85.8	186	60.8	21	17.8	17	4.4	65	39.4	31	9.1
B. Realism-rationalism-relativism oriented																
Politicians/Statesmen	25	15.3	180	45.6	26	8.2	70	22.9	57	48.3	140	36.2	51	30.9	156	45.7
Writers/Poets	5	3.1	10	2.5	2	0.6	12	3.9	8	6.8	17	4.4	11	6.7	25	7.3
Businesspeople	2	1.2	4	1.0	3	0.9	5	1.6	4	3.4	2	0.5	8	4.8	4	1.2
Scientists/Inventors	1	0.6	77	19.5	5	1.6	19	6.2	8	6.8	83	21.4	3	1.8	38	11.1
Public figures[d]	2	1.2	5	1.3	0	0	5	1.6	11	9.3	111	28.7	13	7.9	68	19.9
Famous generals	0	0	16	4.0	4	1.3	4	1.3	3	2.5	10	2.6	3	1.8	10	2.9
Educators/philosophers	2	1.2	5	1.3	0	0	0	0	4	3.4	4	1.0	5	3.0	3	0.9
Artists/Painters	2	1.2	2	0.5	0	0	0	0	0	0	0	0	1	0.6	2	0.6
Musicians	2	1.2	8	2.0	5	1.6	5	1.6	2	1.7	3	0.8	5	3.0	4	1.2
Total	41	25.2	307	77.7	45	14.2	120	39.2	106	82.2	370	95.6	100	60.6	310	90.9

Notes

a The two authors and two research assistants jointly identified the celebrities listed in the table.

b Total number of frequency counts for various kinds of celebrities.

c Many singers in Hong Kong are also movie stars. If so, we define them by the better-known profession. No celebrities were counted twice. The same is true for coding of other celebrities with conflicting roles.

d Public figures in Hong Kong typically include religious people such as Mother Teresa. In China, they include people such as Lei Feng.

superficial and illusory romance (Cheung and Yue 1999). Unsurprisingly, they identify strongly with commercial or hedonic successes and are market driven and media determined when selecting their idols (Leung 1999). This supports the assumption that adolescent idol worship culture in Hong Kong is primarily devoted to pop stars, movie stars, and sports stars for their images of glamour, youthfulness, wealth, and uniqueness (Yue 1999).

Idol worship was examined in a sample of 197 secondary school and university students in Hong Kong (Tseng 2011). Echoing studies showing that Hong Kong students tend to worship the "tri-star figures" (Yue, Wong, and Cheung 2000), both secondary and university students mostly selected music, movie, and sports stars, but university students selected more luminary role models. The findings also support the contention that idolatry decreases with age (White and O'Brien 1999). In addition, idols characterized as having idealism-romanticism-absolutism qualities (e.g., tri-star figures) were significantly more worshipped than those with realism-rationalism-relativism characteristics (e.g., politicians; Table 1.5).

Table 1.5 Paired sample *t*-test comparing orientations regarding idols and role models

Types of idols	Ranking	%	Idol worship M	SD	Model learning M	SD	t-value
A. Idealism-romanticism-absolutism oriented							
Music stars	1	28.9	8.44	1.53	7.60	1.96	5.87**
Movie stars	7	4.8	7.52	1.99	7.37	1.84	.47
Sports stars	10	2.7	8.60	1.45	7.73	1.33	1.94
B. Realism-rationalism-relativism oriented							
Politicians	4	5.5	6.97	2.30	8.23	1.48	−2.88**
Public role models	8	3.9	7.18	2.67	8.14	1.64	−1.60
Writers/poets	9	2.9	7.69	2.89	8.31	1.70	−1.08
Musicians	14	1.3	8.43	1.72	8.43	1.72	/
Businesspeople	10	2.7	8.00	2.14	7.80	2.98	.20
Scientists	16	.9	9.00	1.22	8.20	2.49	.75
Artists/painters	17	.5	6.67	3.51	9.00	1.00	−1.26
Religious figures	15	1.1	9.17	1.33	7.50	3.21	1.54
Educators/philosophers	17	.5	10.00	.00	10.00	.00	/
C. Noncelebrity (relatives)							
Parents	2	18.6	6.75	2.50	8.22	1.66	−5.54**
Other relatives	12	1.8	6.00	2.31	7.70	1.83	−1.68
Siblings	13	1.6	5.00	2.65	5.33	2.65	−.22
D. Noncelebrity (nonrelatives)							
Teachers	3	11.6	5.77	2.64	8.03	1.30	−7.05**
Peers	5	5.2	4.41	2.57	6.79	1.68	−5.71**
Other nonrelatives	6	5.0	5.82	2.84	7.32	1.79	−2.67*
Cartoon characters	17	.5	7.33	1.53	6.67	2.89	.76

Note
*$p < .05$
**$p < .01$

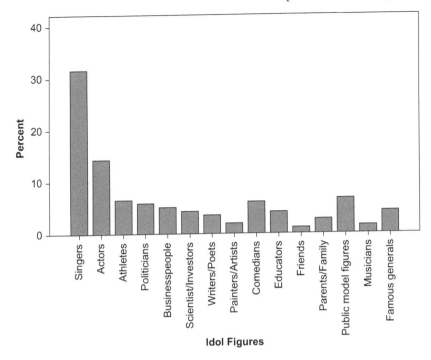

Figure 1.4 Student nominations of idol figures

Noncelebrity relatives and nonrelatives were admired significantly more as role models rather than as idols.

Nearly 35% of the nominated idols were tri-stars, mostly music stars. High school students idolized more tri-stars, whereas university students idolized more luminary figures, implying that university students selected idols because of their charismatic traits or career accomplishments and that high school students selected idols based on glamour or hedonic successes (Yue 1999; Yue and Cheung 2000). Kam (2013) examined a sample of 224 university students in Hong Kong to observe how personality affects selections of favorite celebrities. Consistent with Yue and Cheung (2000a, 2002), Hong Kong students overwhelmingly selected tri-star idols (Figure 1.4).

Hoi-chan Ching (2008) examined 205 students in Hong Kong and found that before the age of 20, they tended to worship media stars, but they admired luminaries across all ages. Those findings support the contention that Hong Kong youth find illusory romance and vainglory fulfillment in media star idols but find enhanced social identity and self-efficacy in luminary role models (Cheung and Yue 2003a, 2003b, 2004; Cheung and Yue 1999, 2000a). In short, Hong Kong students have a worship ethos mainly focused on tri-star figures' youthfulness, wealth, charisma, frivolity, enjoyment, romance, and sex appeal (Cheung and Yue 1999; Yue and Cheung 2000a; Yue et al. 2003). In Mainland China, the idol

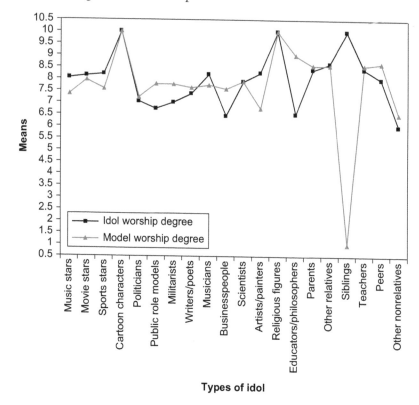

Figure 1.5 Idol worship and model learning for different types of idols

worship ethos emphasizes role models and is oriented toward identification with positive moral values and character (Yue et al. 2003).

As such, Hong Kong highly supports the commercialized entertainment industries (e.g., Chan et al. 1998; Leung 1999), giving the youth culture easy access to entertainment gossip and allowing them to be more easily persuaded by delusional, romantic, and illusory values (Showalter 1997). In contrast, Mainland China students receive a strong moral education and lack exposure to entertainment commercialization. Therefore, they tend to admire more luminary figures as role models for securing healthier self-identity and self-development (Hou et al. 2003; Shen 2001; Yue and Cheung 2002; Wu 2003; Figure 1.5).

Summary

Our study of idol worship in Hong Kong shows that youth tend to idolize "tri-star" figures, perhaps because students are highly aware of society and of people around them. Young women are more likely than young men to have romantic fantasies about handsome and charismatic male idols (Teigen et al. 2000;

Tuval-Mashiach et al. 2008). However, both genders viewed their idols with similar psychological identification, desires for intimacy, and admiration for their accomplishments, which diverges from past findings showing gender differences (e.g., Adams-Price and Greene 1990; Yue and Yan 2009). Further study is needed to examine whether the genders actually differ in the factors that motivate idol worship.

Finally, it is no exaggeration to claim that Hong Kong has been a paradise for adolescents' idol worship, and almost every pop star has his or her own fan club (Cheung and Yue 2003a, 2003b, 2004; Yue and Cheung 2000a; Yue, Wong, and Cheung 2000). The entertainment business is ostensibly responsible for the bombardment of images of pop figures, which represent the major objects of idolizing. Moreover, the entertainment business joins forces with those in the West, Japan, Korea, and other places to amplify its inroads into Hong Kong adolescents' lives. Nevertheless, Hong Kong may be different from other places in the sociocultural context. This difference warrants the examination of idol worship in Hong Kong rather than the simple adoption of knowledge developed from other places. Conversely, the difference justifies the need for testing knowledge originating from research in the West and thereby verifying findings for international reference. This will be discussed more in later sections.

2 Theories and perspectives of idol worship

Three bipolar dimensions differentiate between the worship of idols and of role models: *idealism-realism*, *romanticism-rationalism*, and *absolutism-relativism* (Yue 1999, 2000a, 2000b; Figure 2.1). *Idealism-romanticism-absolutism* (IRA) idol worship indicates that worshippers mystically adore and have romantic love for their idols. *Rationalism-realism-relativism* (RRR) idol worship indicates that admirers see idols as role models suitable for appreciation and emulation. Idol worship may be *person-focused idol worship* (人物为本型偶像崇拜), in which admirers mystically idealize idols as having all desirable attributes, or *attributes-focused idol worship* (特质为本型偶像崇拜), in which admirers appreciate idols for their desirable and imitable attributes.

Idol worship is a unilateral attachment to a vital and overly idealized figure (Fromm 1967). A natural part of human development is that children develop *primary attachments* (初级依恋) through affective parental bonding. As adolescents, they transition to *secondary attachments* (二级依恋), who are often romantic figures (Erikson 1968; Yue and Cheung 2000a).

Adolescents tend to idolize celebrities in the domains of entertainment, sports, politics, science, technology, literature, or art (Yue et al. 2010). The entertainment industry actively persuades fans to see movie stars as having godlike status (Levy 1990). Many adolescents view heavy-metal singers as heroes and fantasy lovers (Jeffrey 1991). Sports stars are also highly attractive in the imaginations and desires of young people (Balswick and Ingoldsby 1982). They admire social luminaries for their merits, social contributions, charisma, or life philosophies (Yue et al. 2010).

Various theories have been offered to explain adolescent idol worship. Freud (1925) identified the importance of childhood development through identification with suitable parental figures. Blos (1967) and Josselson (1991) argued that as adolescents search for identity and progress toward intimacy with significant others, they need idols to serve as role models for establishing values and preparing for adulthood (Erikson 1968). Idols also provide a secure base while the ego grows (Pleiss and Feldhusen 1995).

Bandura (1977) argued that imitation and role modeling are essential for developing appropriate social skills. Imitation and role modeling includes four steps: attention, retention, motor reproduction, and motivation. Individuals

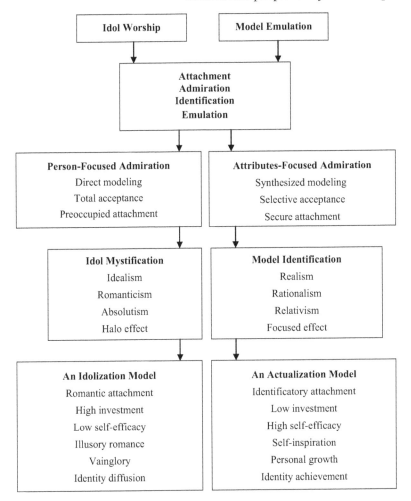

Figure 2.1 Difference between idol worship and model emulation (Yue 2001)

follow the four steps when they observe whether behaviors are rewarded or punished, acceptable or unacceptable (Yue and Cheung 2000a).

Psychological theories of idol worship

Several theories have been offered to explain idol worship. *Psychoanalytical theory* posits that appropriate parental figures are essential for child development. If parents are good models, the child has a secure base for ego development (Pleiss and Feldhusen 1995). If parents provide an insecure base, the child is likely to be anxious and prone to panic and to display immature ego development. Alternatively, children must evolve identities that imitate and endorse their parents but are distinct from them. As such, idols may provide the secure base required for ego development. Consequently, idols may help adolescents transition from their original parental attachments to closer and romantic attachments to significant others (Erikson 1968; Freud 1951). Model effects appear to increase as children identify with their heroes (Hamilton and Darling 1996).

Individuation theory maintains that idols can meet needs for identification and intimacy essential for adolescent ego development (e.g., Josselson 1991). Adolescents lack firm personal identities and must discover their identities as part of natural development (Marcia 1980). By identifying with role models or idols, they reinforce their values and learn to adopt adult roles.

Secondary attachment theory proposes that idols fulfill instrumental needs for emotional bonding. Adolescents form imaginary relationships with distant figures, such as fantasized friendships or romantic relationships with pop music stars and movie actors (Davidson 1983; Erikson 1968; Yue and Cheung 2000a, 2000b). The idol is not the true focus of attachment but is instead the object of fantasy, mystification, and idealized attributes, with imagined closeness or intimacy as a friend or romantic partner (Fromm 1967). Secondary attachments may be *romantic attachments* or *identificatory attachments* (Adams-Price and Greene 1990). Men tend to have identificatory attachments to male celebrities according to instrumentality (e.g., potency), whereas women tend to have romantic attachments to male celebrities according to expressivity (e.g., amity). Similarly, fans might fantasize about becoming celebrities themselves if they become romantic partners with their idols. Hence, adolescent idol worship is generally identificatory romantic attachment to achieve identity and intimacy. The attachment is a way to facilitate individuation from parents (Winnicott 1965).

Social learning theory maintains that imitation and role modeling are vital for developing suitable social skills (Bandura 1986). Behavior modeling proceeds sequentially through the four steps of attention, retention, motor reproduction, and motivation. Adolescents learn to regulate their behaviors by observing how behaviors are rewarded or punished. For example, low-achieving students who doubted their ability to learn progressed when they were encouraged to identify with models who were once low achievers but successfully persevered (Schunk and Hanson 1985). Similarly, celebrity modeling can develop future aspirations that form the basis for identities. Nevertheless, although identification and imitation are similar, children's dispositional traits will determine whether their idolization leads to identification rather than imitation (Feshbach and Weiner 1986).

Compensation perspective on idol worship

Compensation theory suggests that idol worship may function as compensation for deficits in psychosocial development, cognitive development, attachment, companionship, social networking, and romantic relationships as well as other weaknesses. For example, idol worship may appear to represent one's fantasized attachment to remote figures (Engle and Kasser 2005), imaginary companionship

(Seiffge-Krenke 1997), entertainment (McCutcheon et al. 2003), reflection of value or expectancy (Singer et al. 1993), deficiency in psychosocial development (Giles 2000; Seiffge-Krenke 1997), deficiency in cognitive development (Seiffge-Krenke 1997), and absorption and addiction (McCutcheon et al. 2003). Hence, when the worshipper has a surplus in something, the worshipper will choose to worship something else. The compensation theory has been useful in identifying fragile or low self-esteem, weak social alliance, and monotonous life experience as determinants of idol worship (Jenson 1992).

Compensatory and compatibility perspectives of idol worship

Based on previous studies and theoretical propositions, two general and contrasting perspectives have emerged to explain idolatrous behaviors around the world, particularly for adolescents. The *compensatory perspective of idol worship* (偶像崇拜补偿论) regards celebrity worshippers as absorbed, addicted, obsessive individuals who lack meaningful relationships (McCutcheon et al. 2002; Meloy 1998; Szymanski 1977; Willis 1972). Their absorption compromises their identity structure (Cheng 2017) so that they devote their "total attention, involving a full commitment of available perceptual, motoric, imaginative, and ideational resources to a unified representation of the attentional object" (Tellegen and Atkinson 1974, p. 274). They have lost a sense of reality and are overcome with erroneous beliefs that they maintain special ties with the celebrity. Extreme celebrity worship features obsessive-compulsive and even delusional symptoms (Cheng 2017) in which worshippers are deeply motivated to learn about and achieve closeness to the admired celebrity.

The Celebrity Attitude Scale (CAS) is useful for measuring celebrity worship (Maltby, Houran, Lange, Ashe, and McCutcheon 2002; Maltby et al. 2001; McCutcheon et al. 2002). It contains 23 items to identify three grades of celebrity worship:

- *Entertainment-social* celebrity worship is about entertainment and socializing. Sample items are "I know I will have a good time watching, reading, or listening to my favorite celebrity" and "I enjoy being with others who like my favorite celebrity."
- *Intense-personal* celebrity worship is about intensity and compulsiveness. Sample items are "When something good happens to my favorite celebrity, I feel like it happened to me" and "I frequently think about my favorite celebrity, even when I don't want to."
- *Borderline-pathological* celebrity worship is about uncontrollable behaviors and fantasies. Sample items are "If I were lucky enough to meet my favorite celebrity, and he/she asked me to do something illegal, I would probably do it" and "If someone gave me several thousand dollars to do with as I please, I would consider spending it on a personal possession (such as a napkin or paper plate) once used by my favorite celebrity."

Individuals who score high on the CAS scale have potential emotional and psychological difficulties, such as obsessive concerns about body image (Maltby et al. 2005) and a higher likelihood of seeking cosmetic surgery (Swami et al. 2009). They tend to be sensation seeking and cognitively rigid and have diffused identity and poor interpersonal boundaries (Houran et al. 2005). They may show other psychological difficulties, such as extreme religiosity (Maltby et al. 2002), poor coping styles (Maltby et al. 2004), narcissism (Maltby et al. 2003; Maltby et al. 2004), fantasy proneness and dissociation (Maltby et al. 2006), and skewed attributional style and self-esteem (Sheridan, North, Maltby, and Gillett 2007).

Celebrity worshippers who have intense-personal and borderline-pathological interest in celebrities are likely to experience mental problems such as depression, anxiety, social dysfunction, and negative affect (Maltby et al. 2004; Maltby et al. 2001); dissociation (Maltby et al. 2006); addictive tendencies (McCutcheon et al. 2002); criminal tendencies (Melton 2000; Sheridan et al. 2007); stalking behaviors (McCutcheon, Scott, Aruguete, and Parker 2006); and compulsive buying (Reeves et al. 2012). However, celebrity worship has not been linked with Axis I or Axis II psychiatric diagnoses (Sansone and Sansone 2014).

In contrast, the *compatibility perspective of idol worship* (偶像崇拜相容论) suggests that celebrity worship includes parasocial and social interactions that complement self-development (Yue and Cheung 2000a, 2000b; Yue et al. 2000). For example, identification with comedians causes parasocial relationship experiences that enhance self-esteem and social skills (Yue, Wong, & Cheung, 2000). Celebrity worshippers seem to form social relations based on behavior learned through parasocial interactions (Berger 1986; Berger and Calabrese 1975).

Over the past 20 years, fans have formed self-identify and self-esteem by idolizing the tri-stars and other celebrity figures, but adolescents gain the most benefits when they idolize luminary figures rather than tri-star figures (e.g., Cheung and Yue 2000, 2003a, 2003b; Yue and Cheung 2000a, 2000b; Yue, Wong, and Cheung 2000). Yue and Cheung developed the 26-item Idol Worship Questionnaire (IWQ) to measure idol worship, which includes measures for the following:

- *Identification-emulation.* Fans experience personal growth by identifying role models for learning and emulation (Calvert, Murray, and Conger 2004) and for identifying themselves as unique, self-sufficient, and separate from the idol (Greene and Adams-Price 1990; Stevens 2010). Thus, the idol is an inspirational role model.
- *Attachment-romanticization.* Fans feel close affiliation, as if the idol were a powerful, amiable, and protective friend or family member (Cotterell 1992; Larose and Boivin 1998; North, Desborough, and Shars 2005). The attachment may be illusory, fantasized infatuation (Cheung and Yue 2004;

Greene and Adams-Price 1990) in which fans imagine that they and the idol are mutually entangled extensions of one another (Engle and Kasser 2005). The worshipper then loses his or her sense of self.

- *Idealization-mystification.* The idol is perceived as having godlike power and omnipotence. Idealization is most commonly manifested in religious worship in which the idol is the master and the worshipper is the deferential, unquestioning slave (Porter 1988; Regnerus 2003). Thus, internalization is unlikely.
- *Consumption-commitment.* Capitalist, market, entertainment, and media industries now encourage fan obsessiveness to commodify celebrity worship (Schultze et al. 1991; Stevens 2010). The idol is no longer a person and becomes an object for fetishism and consumption (Bowman 1998).

Our studies generally show that identification with and idealization of admired idols is positively associated with higher self-esteem and self-efficacy and negatively associated with social anxiety and attachment problems. However, romanticization of and attachment to admired idols are associated with lower self-esteem and self-efficacy and greater social anxiety and attachment problems (Cheung and Yue 2000, 2003a, 2003b; Yue and Cheung 2000a, 2000b; Yue, Wong, and Cheung 2000).

We surveyed 1,095 students attending secondary schools in Hong Kong and Shenzhen to observe whether students identified with and emulated role models for achievement-oriented purposes (Yue, Cheung, and Wong 2010). We found that achievement-oriented worshippers frequently identified the celebrity Andy Lau[1] as a target associated with psychological gravitations and desires to glorify, idealize, identify with, and emulate a role model. The study will be discussed in greater detail in the following section.

In short, I discuss above two contrasting perspectives on understanding idolatrous behaviors in modern times. Apart from their differences in theoretical propositions, they also differ in measurements. That is, the three original components of celebrity—entertainment and socializing, personalizing, and obsession—are very likely to tap a single dimension of involvement. Hence, they may maintain very high intercorrelations, making them redundant to each other. To assuage the redundancy problem, reorganizing the items of celebrity worship into distinctive dimensions is necessary in order to retain most information in the items. A promising way is to restructure the measure into attachment, romanticization, idealization, and consumption to resemble the commitment dimensions of idol worship. In such a way, idolatrous behaviors, whether for celebrities or noncelebrities, can be examined in a more comprehensive way. Conceivably, differences between the present measures of idol worship and celebrity worship may be attributable to cultural differences in the origin of the measures. With the minimization of differences due to conceptualization, further research can better assess the remaining distinctiveness in idol worship and celebrity worship. This will be discussed in later paragraphs.

Li Yuchun[2]: The grassroots girl who became a pop queen

In recent years, a pop singer called Li Yuchun (李宇春) gained huge popularity in China. Miss Li was born in Chengdu in 1984 and received no professional training in singing until she participated in the Supergirl Contest (超女; a talent show similar to *American Idol*) in 2005. Li won the contest partly owing to her boyish appearance and clothing style. She has been referred to as "Brother Chun" (春哥) ever since and is generally called "handsome" instead of "pretty."

Brother Chun has become more than the winner of a talent show; she has become a cultural phenomenon. She has also iconized herself to her fans as a symbol of aspiration and inspiration for grassroots youngsters. Specifically, to those young dreamers who want to become successful pop singers without proper training or qualifications, Brother Chun represents a super success that could come from one's own diligence and determination; to those who want to speak or act as they like, Brother Chun is a super role model as to how to please oneself before pleasing others; to those who want to succeed without special backgrounds, Brother Chun is a perfect example of succeeding on one's own merits.

In brief, Li Yuchun is not a super idol to her followers; she is a super role model.

As Duong (2009) nicely summarizes: "Li Yuchun was totally the opposite of what almost all female Chinese pop singers were like. She was 1.74 meters tall; kept short hair; wore pants and T-shirts, and no makeup; sang songs written for male singers such as 'In my heart there's only you, never her' and sang in a bass voice, danced in a Ricky Martin style. Li Yuchun's stardom led to a huge dispute on the tomboy trend and sexuality, because it challenged the conventional Chinese criteria for feminine aesthetics and traditional gender norms among Chinese youths" (p. 33).

Source: Duong, Thanh Nga. 2009. *China's Supergirl Show: Democracy and Female Empowerment among Chinese Youth* (master's thesis). Centre for East and South East Asian Studies, Lund University, Lund, Sweden.

Role model emulation

Worthy role models can help young people develop and learn positive behavior, skills, and beliefs (Bandura 1986; Berger 1977; Field 1981; Rosenthal and Zimmerman 1978).

Role model learning particularly encourages students to develop their talents and learn new skills (Bandura 1986; Schunk 1987). For example, low-achieving students who indicated doubt about their ability to learn were shown to benefit by identifying with a role model who had similar doubts, persevered, and was eventually successful (Schunk and Hanson 1985). In addition, modeling after a celebrity figure can help students form future aspirations and identity.

In response to promotions from the entertainment industry, young people in Hong Kong are fondest of tri-star figures (e.g., Leung 1999; Yue and Cheung 2002; Yue, Cheung, and Wong 2010). In China, by contrast, the government strives to encourage identification with heroism and altruism. Consequently, young people are more attracted to public and governmental role models, such as self-sacrificing political heroes, war martyrs, and accomplished scholars typically devoted to social duty, even at personal risk.

One noteworthy exemplar is Lei Feng,[3] an altruistic young soldier who died while serving in the military. His heroism has been well publicized for decades, and he is considered a suitable model for young Chinese people.[4] His humble, plain, and ordinary personality, his simple lifestyle, and his altruistic dedication sharply contrast with the image of pop stars.

China has become increasingly open to the world since the early 1980s. Although Chinese youth have been exposed to pop stars from the West, Japan, Taiwan, and Hong Kong, they continue to idolize political figures, public models, and accomplished scholars as before, and Lei Feng remains a top role model because of the government's promotional efforts.

Cheung and Yue (2003b) conducted a telephone survey of 833 teenagers in Hong Kong to explore the influence of idols on identity development. The survey revealed that illusory romance, reification, and vainglory orientation in idol worship predicted deficient identity achievement. In another survey of 1,641 secondary school students in Hong Kong and Mainland China, participants who identified luminaries as role models were more likely to report having self-efficacy; participants who adored star idols were less likely to report having self-efficacy (Cheung and Yue 2003a). A study of junior middle school students showed that students who worshipped and learned from idols tended to have favorable self-concepts (Wang and Li 2013). Those studies offered empirical evidence that parasocial interaction contributes to identity development (Cheung and Yue 2003b; Yue and Cheung 2000a, 2000b; Yue et al. 2010).

A study of 1,095 secondary school students in Hong Kong and Shenzhen was conducted to experimentally prime the effects of idol worship. In the *glamour-frame condition*, participants were primed to see an idol as having perfect, mystical, or ideological characteristics. In the *achievement-frame condition*, they were primed to emulate and identify with prosocial and virtuous behaviors (Yue et al. 2010). The idol was the eminent local artist Andy Lau. Students in the achievement-frame condition indicated significantly greater desires to emulate, idealize, and attach to Andy Lau than did students in the glamour-frame condition. The findings suggest that priming can cause students to perceive star idols as role models.

The study revealed that idol worship was consistently higher in the achievement-frame condition than in the glamour-frame condition across all measured items. Hence, the achievement frame was more conducive for increasing idol

Table 2.1 Means by frames and locations

Idol worship indicator	Hong Kong		Shenzhen	
	Glamour frame (n = 430)	Achievement frame (n = 328)	Glamour frame (n = 182)	Achievement frame (n = 155)
Vain glorification	28.9	33.6	25.8	28.6
Idealization	29.3	35.2*	26.0	34.9*
Identification	43.5	47.0	56.4	57.5
Emulation	37.3	43.4*	49.3	56.4
Attachment	45.9	48.2	54.4	65.6*

Note
*$p < .05$

worship (Table 2.1). Moreover, the multivariate test indicated that five desired characteristics of idol worship differ significantly between the achievement and glamour conditions ($F = 6.509$, $p < .001$). The findings imply that greater exposure to achievement framing rather than glamour framing could reduce idol worship and encourage dedication to role models.

The findings also indicated that priming encouraged greater idealization (8.9 vs. 5.9) and attachment (11.2 vs. 2.3) for the youth of Shenzhen than for the youth of Hong Kong. Overall, the multivariate test showed that framing caused significant differences in the five dimensions of idol worship ($F = 2.643$, $p = .022$).

As Table 2.2 shows, the priming effects were apparent in all five dimensions of idol worship among the young men. Among the young women, the priming effects were salient only in the idealization dimension. Accordingly, for the young men, all aspects of idol worship were significantly higher for the achievement frame than for the glamour frame. In contrast, for the young women, only idealization was significantly higher. Overall, framing caused the multivariate test of the differential effects on the five dimensions of idol worship to endorse significant differentials ($F = 1.987$, $p = .078$). Particularly, framing caused the difference identification (7.8 vs. −1.1, $F = 4.790$, $p = .029$) to be significantly higher in young men than in young women.

Table 2.2 Means by frames and sexes

Idol worship indicator	Young men		Young women	
	Glamour frame (n = 297)	Achievement frame (n = 252)	Glamour frame (n = 276)	Achievement frame (n = 227)
Vain glorification	25.1	33.2*	28.3	29.8
Idealization	26.3	36.1*	26.6	33.3*
Identification	46.1	53.9*	49.1	48.2
Emulation	40.9	50.3*	41.4	45.8
Attachment	46.5	55.0*	49.1	54.3

Note
*$p < .05$

The findings also indicated that priming caused greater differences in terms of idealization (8.9 vs. 5.9) and attachment (11.2 vs. 2.3) for the youth in Shenzhen than for the youth in Hong Kong. Overall, a multivariate test showed that framing caused significant differences in the five dimensions of idol worship ($F = 2.643, p = .022$).

Among young men, the priming effects were apparent in all five dimensions of idol worship. In contrast, among young women, the priming effects were significant only in the idealization component. Accordingly, all components were significantly higher for the achievement frame than for the glamour frame among young men. In contrast, only idealization was significantly higher among young women. Overall, framing caused the multivariate test of effects on the five components of idol worship to display significant differentials ($F = 1.987, p = .078$). Particularly, framing caused significantly higher differences in identification for the young men (7.8 vs. $-1.1, F = 4.790, p = .029$).

Students exposed to achievement framing regarding Andy Lau showed stronger achievement-oriented idolatry (AOI) than did students exposed to the glamour frame (glamour-oriented idolatry, GOI), which supports the assumption that star idols would be more admired if their personal achievements were emphasized. As such, superbly glamorous and charismatic star idols can be transformed into role models for encouraging aspirations and self-determination. Role modeling has been shown to increase identification with observed characters (Lesser 1974) and to help young people identify their potential roles (Gash and Conway 1997). Training programs have been shown to help children identify with the appropriate gender (Gash and Morgan 1993; Gash, Morgan, and Sugure 1993).

Priming had different effects on students in Hong Kong and Mainland China. In China, students are taught moral dedication and patriotic orientations regarding heroes and socialist goals. Consequently, Shenzhen students were more responsive to achievement priming about Andy Lau. Mainland China leaders have called for more role model education (Xue 1997). Regarding gender differentials, young men were more responsive than young women to Andy Lau's achievements, which implies that young men would be more likely to transform star idols into role models.

The study implies that AOI programs should be developed to enhance critical thinking, to encourage truth seeking, and to attenuate paranormal and absolute beliefs about popular idols and authoritarian figures (e.g., Halpern 1998; MacPhee, Kreutzer, and Pritz 1994). The Hong Kong government requires that secondary schools include liberal studies that foster critical thinking. AOI should be a component of liberal studies to foster critical thinking and to transform glamour-based idol worship to achievement-based idol worship.

Summary

In summary, the compensatory perspective of idolatry holds that idolatrous behaviors are generally symptomatic of problems/deficits in psychosocial and cognitive development and resources whereas the compatibility perspective of idolatry maintains that idolatrous behaviors are indicative of needs/motives of positive psychosocial development. Deficits in cognitive development may occur in one's egocentrism or failure to take account of others' and societal perspectives, which results in one's overemphasis on uniqueness and imagination (Seiffge-Krenke 1997). Apart from the individual's own deficiency, inadequacy in social relationships and other life experiences would be a concern for seeking compensation (Jenson 1992). For instance, idol worship has appeared to stem from inadequate attachment to parents (Giles and Maltby 2004), absence of close and secure relationships (Giles and Maltby 2004), inadequacy in social complexity and cognitive flexibility (Maltby et al. 2004), and cognitive deficits in creativity, critical thinking, need for cognition, spatial ability, and crystallized intelligence (McCutcheon et al. 2003). In contrast, when young people identify their favored idols as role models, they may develop self-efficacy and enhance self-identity by learning from role models who have achieved fame, but ideally, they should learn from instrumental, practical, and realistic role models rather than overly idealized, fantasized star idols (Adams-Price and Greene 1990; Fromm 1967). Moreover, school-based programs should be developed to enhance critical thinking, to encourage truth seeking, and to attenuate paranormal and absolute beliefs about popular idols and authoritarian figures.

Turning star idols into role models

Over the years of my studying adolescent idol worship behaviors in Chinese societies, I have been frequently invited to address at various conferences and seminars about how to help young people to engage in critical and constructive idolatry. The answer I give is **to turn star idols into role models**.

Specifically, I would invite young people to search for dispositional identification with their admired idols rather than simply adoring their glamour and wealth. In so doing, they will find virtues and strength in their favored idols. Besides, I would also invite parents and schoolteachers to give up their prejudiced views against kids' favored idols and to look for desirable dispositional traits and virtues that could be used for enhancing their positive self-development.

In fact, many schools in China has taken my advice seriously by setting up "idol sharing days" for teachers/parents to discuss with students why they would idolize a given celebrity or noncelebrity in their life and how they could benefit from it. This not only helps students to communicate openly with teachers/parents why they admire their favored idols and what they mean to them, it also helps teachers/parents to learn to empathize with their students/children as to how to look for inspirational figures during adolescence. Collectively, teachers and students may discuss, for the first time, and peacefully and rationally, the potential benefits of idol worship in students' life. And this has never been done before!

To turn star idols into role models, it all depends on how willingly teachers/parents can give up their own prejudiced views against the star idols favored by students, and how wisely teachers/parents can use these star idols for positive self-development for students.

My study on Andy Lau (劉德華) set up an example for development of such programs in China.

Source: Changing idols as an example—Dr. Xiaodong Xiao talks about idols—model education. Retrieved from http://www.jinyueya.com/magazine/5919665.htm

3 Comparing and verifying absorption-addiction idolatry and identification-emulation idolatry

Hong Kong is a paradise for popular culture (e.g., Cheung and Yue 2003a, 2003b; Yue and Cheung 2000a, 2000b; Yue, Cheung, and Wong 2010), with a renowned free-market system that popularizes idols and celebrities. Because Hong Kong is the hub and bridge of Chinese and Western cultures, images of idols and celebrities swamp Hong Kong media. Hong Kong has the modern technology to publicize celebrities and encourage celebrity worship, as in the rest of the developed world (Hoover and Stokes 2003).

Hong Kong's culture and structure are conducive to idol worship among the young, who tend to be oriented toward laissez-faire socioeconomics, risk taking, resistance to conventional norms, innovative fashion, and social mobility (Lai and Bryam 2003; Lam, Stewart, and Ho 2001; Law, Zhang, and Leung 2000; Tse 2007). Those characteristics promote the worship of unconventional celebrities with strong youth appeal.

Cheung and Yue (2018) proposed two conceptual models to explain differences in idol worship (Table 3.1). *Absorption-addiction idolatry* (AAI) describes obsessive idolatry. *Identification-emulation idolatry* (IEI) describes imagined mutual closeness with enhanced or idealized attributes of idolized figures.

Absorption indicates "total attention, involving a full commitment of available perceptual, motoric, imaginative, and ideational resources to form a unified representation of the attentional object" (Tellegent and Atkinson 1974, p. 274). As such, absorption indicates total attention leading to a heightened sense of reality. AAI can lead worshippers to erroneously believe that they share special connections with their idols. They then seek proximity to idols, perceiving them as having mystical glamour, wealth, and physical attractiveness. Such absorption may cause addictive behavior patterns along with obsessive-compulsive and even delusional behaviors. The celebrity becomes the center of meaning.

The AAI model indicates three motivations for celebrity attachments. That is, worshippers seek to fulfill *entertainment-social, intense-personal*, and *borderline-pathological* needs (McCutcheon, Ashe, Houran, and Maltby 2003). Worshippers seeking to fulfill *entertainment-social* needs tend to admire and follow celebrities to enjoy their talent and to provide a source of social interaction,

Table 3.1 Summary of contrasting characteristics of the AAI and the IEI (Cheung and Yue 2018)

Idolatry features	Malty and McCutcheon's model	Yue and Cheung's model
Conceptualization	Absorption-addiction model of idolatry (AAI)	Identification-emulation model of idolatry (IEI)
Focus	Glamour-based adoration: fame, grandeur, wealth, physical attractiveness	Charisma-based admiration: personality, talents, personal accomplishments
Nature	Pathological, additive	Developmental, normal
Type	Mostly star idols, e.g., pop singers, movie stars, sports stars, fashion models, and DJs	Mostly luminaries: e.g., scientists, philosophers, writers, businesspeople, and statesmen
Role	Compensates for core self-evaluation (Judge et al. 1997)	Complements core self-evaluation (Turner 1993)
Consequence	Weakens core self-evaluations	Strengthens core self-evaluations
Measures	Celebrity attitude scale (CAS) • Entertainment-social • Intense-personal • Borderline-pathological	Idol worship questionnaire (IWQ) • Glorification-idealization • Identification-emulation • Attachment-consumption

such as gossiping about celebrities with friends. Worshippers seeking to fulfill *intense-personal* needs tend to have strong, compulsive, obsessive feelings about favorite celebrities. Worshippers seeking to fulfill *borderline-pathological* needs tend to show uncontrollable behaviors and fantasies about celebrities. Thus, the AAI depicts celebrity worship in terms of involvement, progressing from absorption to filling personal emptiness to addiction (Maltby, Day, McCutcheon, Gillett, Houran, and Ashe 2004).

Excessive idol worship can have significant negative effects on mental health, including (1) depression, anxiety, social dysfunction, and negative affect (Maltby, McCutcheon, Gillet, Houran, and Ashe 2004); (2) dissociation (Maltby, McCutcheon, Houran, and Ashe 2006); (3) addiction (McCutcheon, Lang, and Houran 2002); (4) criminality (Melton 2000; Sheridan, North, Maltby, and Gillet 2007); (5) stalking behaviors (McCutcheon, Scott, Aruguete, and Parker 2006); and (6) compulsive buying (Reeves, Baker, and Truluck 2012). Intense-personal and borderline-pathological interests are most likely to be associated with mental difficulties, but empirical evidence is lacking for associations with Axis I or Axis II psychiatric diagnoses (Sansone and Sansone 2014).

An ardent fan's tragic story

Yang Lijuan (杨丽娟; 1978–) became obsessed with Andy Lau (刘德华) when she was 16 after dreaming about him. She lived in Lanzhou (兰州),

Gansu (甘肃), with her father, Qinji Yang (杨勤冀), a former school-teacher, and her mother, a disabled housewife. Lijuan became so preoccupied with fan club activities that she dropped out of school. Her father initially objected but eventually fully supported her, although he feared that she might be possessed by a devil. He spent their family savings to finance trips to Lau's concerts, and he even sold part of his kidney to meet the ever-increasing demands.

In March 2007, the three went to Hong Kong to attend a fan club birthday party for Lau. Both parents were thrilled when Lijuan finally met Lau. She had her photo taken with her idol and then asked to see him privately for 10 minutes. Her father contacted Lau's agent to try to arrange a private meeting, but Lau bluntly refused. Qinji Yang wrote a letter of protest and then drowned himself at sea in Tsim Sha Tsui (尖沙嘴), hoping that Lau would sympathize and fulfill Lijuan's wish. When Lau heard about the incident, he published a letter calling for fans to stop such irrational fan worship.

Lijuan regrets that her idolization led to her father's death. She advises: "Don't be a crazy fan. After all, Andy Lau is not worth wasting my time or yours."

Source: http://evchk.wikia.com/wiki/%E6%A5%8A%E9%BA%97%E5%A8%9F

Identification-emulation idolatry

The *identification-emulation idolatry* model indicates that worshippers identify with enhanced or idealized attributes of idolized figures and an imagined sense of closeness (Yue and Cheung 2000; Yue et al. 2010). IEI considers idolatry to be a normal part of identity formation, with potential benefits for enhancing core self-evaluations. In the IEI model, fans look to admired celebrities as inspirational role models for self-growth. They admire celebrities' charisma, talents, and personal accomplishments as guidelines to be emulated. The IEI model indicates that fans seek to fulfill their desires for *attachment, consumption, identification, idealization,* and *romanticization* (Adams-Price and Greene 1990; Cheung and Yue 2000; Yue 1999).

Attachment indicates that worshippers feel closely affiliated with idols, viewing them as powerful, amiable, and protective friends or family members (Larose and Boivin 1998; North, Desborough, and Shars 2005). *Consumption* is the result of capitalist, market, entertainment, and media forces that promote commodification (Stevens 2010) in which idols become objectified, fetishist, materialistic commodities rather than real people (Bowman 1998; Schultze et al. 1991). *Idealization* is commonly manifested in religious worship, in which worshippers show slave/master deference to idols sanctified as having unparalleled, unquestionable, omnipotent, godlike power (Porter 1988; Regnerus 2003). *Identification* means that worshippers look to idols as role models for learning, emulation, and personal growth (Calvert, Murray, and Conger 2004), but they maintain their self-worth so that they grow personally, separately from the idol (Adams-Price and Green 1990). Thus, the worshipper develops unique and sufficient self-identity (Stevens 2010). *Romanticization* indicates that worshippers have an infatuated, fantasized love for the idol (Cheung and Yue 2004; Adams-Price and Green 1990), imagining they are mutually and mystically entangled extensions of one another (Engle and Kasser 2005).

Illusory romance, reification, and glorification of idols have been shown to predict lower identity achievement (Cheung and Yue 2003a), while identification and emulation have been shown to predict higher self-esteem and identity formation (Yue, Cheung and Wong 2010). Star idols are associated with idealism, romanticism, and absolutism; role models are associated with realism, rationalism, and relativism (Cheung and Yue 2000). Hong Kong youth tend to admire both idols and role models. Their idols are associated with idealism, romanticism, and absolutism, and their role models are associated with realism, rationalism, and relativism (Yue and Cheung 2000).

A study of 1,095 secondary school students in Hong Kong and Shenzhen focused on the psychological mechanisms involved in achievement-oriented idol worship (Yue, Cheung, and Wong 2010). Participants who were inclined to adopt achievement-oriented idolatry rather than glamour-oriented idolatry were more likely to glorify, idealize, identify with, emulate, and attach to idols.

Jack Ma's "Feng Qingyang" legacy

On November 3, 2017, Jack Ma, the founder of Alibaba, released his first movie, *Gong Shou Road* (《功守道》). Although the movie is about martial arts, audiences were surprised when Faye Wong (王菲)[1] and Jack Ma (马云) sang the theme song "Feng Qingyang" (风清扬) together. Faye Wong has been one of the most popular singers in China and Hong Kong for the past 20 years, but Jack Ma has never claimed to be a singer.

Ma has been a die-hard fan of Faye Wong for many years. After he initiated the Double 11 Shopping Festival,[2] he repeatedly invited her to sing for the event. She declined for three years but accepted in 2017. He chose the song they sang together, about Ma's favorite character from Jin Yong's (金庸)[3] novel *Laughter and Pride* (《笑傲江湖》).

The duet was thus a combined tribute to Jack Ma's favorite idols: Faye Wong and Jin Yong. Ma summarized the all-encompassing feelings inherent in fandom: "I will become you when I admire you."

Of course, the chorus was costly for Jack Ma, costing 1.6 billion RMB!

Although it has been useful to examine studies of conceptualizations regarding idol worship in this chapter, researchers have failed to examine the relationship between the AAI and IEI models discussed. Thus, research is needed to clarify similarities and dissimilarities between modalities of idolatry. The conceptual differences might be explored as pathological over identification contrasted with normal wishful identification (Cheng 2017), or identification in which fans believe that they are similar to their idols (Stever 2009).

Verification of AAI and IEI

Clarification of the relationship and differentials between AAI and IEI is crucial for understanding causes and consequences. Both significantly affect youth development, behaviors, and lifestyles; they affect the economy through consumption and the social order through delinquency and substance abuse (End et al. 2002; Houran, Navik, and Zerrusen 2005; Reeves et al. 2012; Sheridan, North, Maltby, and Gillett 2007).

Celebrity worshippers are prone to form or join fan clubs that reinforce their attachments (End et al. 2002; Ferris 2001; Turner and Scherman 1996). Fan club members are more likely to exhibit AAI and to show deviant behavior, such as stalking and drug abuse, indicating absorption and addiction (Ferris 2001; North et al. 2005).

To verify these conceptual differences, Cheung and Yue (2018) studied a sample of 1,310 secondary school and university students in Hong Kong. They used the Celebrity Attitude Scale (CAS), which includes 23 items to measure AAI at three levels (Maltby, Day, McCutcheon, Gillett, Houran, and Ashe 2004). A sample item: "My friends and I like to discuss what my favorite celebrity has done." To measure IEI idol worship, they use the Idol Worship Questionnaire, which includes 26 items measuring 10 dimensions (Cheung and Yue 2011). The measure has evolved over a decade through qualitative and statistical analyses of data collections from Chinese societies (Yue and Cheung 2000a, 2000b, 2002; Yue et al. 2010). A sample item:

"I wish I could become the kind of person I idolize."

Table 3.2 Means and standard deviations

Variable	Scoring	M	SD
Age	years	17.7	3.4
Female	0–100	49.3	50.0
Fan club membership	0–100	21.6	41.2
Idol worship			
Identification	0–100	58.1	22.7
Attachment	0–100	54.7	25.4
Romanticization	0–100	29.5	26.7
Idealization	0–100	41.2	26.5
Consumption	0-100	35.5	25.0
Celebrity worship			
Entertainment/socializing	0–100	48.5	21.1
Personalizing	0–100	39.8	22.4
Obsession (pathological)	0–100	31.0	21.8

Structural equation modeling showed that all models fit the data quite well (Table 3.2 and Table 3.3; Cheung and Yue 2018). Notably, the standardized root-mean-square residual was less than .05, the root-mean-square error of approximation was less than .07, and the comparative goodness-of-fit index (CFI) approached .95, even with a large number (38) of input variables (Marsh et al. 2004). Nevertheless, Model 2, which specified two second-order factors, was the most parsimonious in terms of the Bayesian information criterion (270963 < 271107 or 271053). Moreover, Model 3, which identified only one second-order factor, yielded a noticeably poorer fit than Models 1 and 2 (CFI = .941 < .951 or .948; Cheung and Rensvold 2002). Hence, Models 1 and 2 were preferable to Model 3 for differentiating between idol worship and celebrity worship factors.

Factor loadings were adequately high on all the factors of idol worship or celebrity worship, implying that all five first-order factors of idol worship, three first-order factors of celebrity worship, and two second-order factors based on the first-order factors attained substantial factor loadings or convergent validity. The discriminant validity of the celebrity worship factor was lower than that of the idol worship factor. In all, the factors of idol worship and celebrity worship were identifiable with favorable structural validity, convergent validity, and discriminant validity. Herein, structural validity meant the identification of the second-order factors of idol worship and celebrity worship.

Finally, fan club membership and female gender had significant effects, suggesting that fan club membership has an expected significant positive effect on the second-order factor of celebrity worship ($\beta = .259$) but not that of idol worship ($\beta = .130$). Female gender had a significant effect on both idol worship and celebrity worship ($\beta = .276, -.431$), but age had no significant effect on idol worship or celebrity worship, although the effect was in the expected negative direction.

Table 3.3 Standardized factor loadings estimated for Model 2

Factor/indicator	Trait	Method
First-order factor		
Idol worship Questionnaire (IWQ)		
Identification (first-order)		
I wish that I could become the kind of person whom I idolize	.379	.479
I see my idol as a role model to my personal development	.552	.424
Whenever I think of my idol, I cannot help feeling inspired	.945	.416
Attachment (first-order)		
I wish that I would become a friend to my idol	.512	.428
I dream that one day, I could get acquainted with my idol and talk with him freely	.616	.399
I always feel that my idols are as amiable as my elder brothers or sisters	.695	.395
Romanticization (first-order)		
I wish that I would become the lover to my idol	.715	.405
I consider my idol as my dream romantic partner	.787	.412
I dream that my idol would like me as well	.624	.431
Idealization (first-order)		
I believe that my idol is the most perfect person in the world	.730	.425
I feel that my idol is irreplaceable by anyone else	.842	.384
I feel that my idol is the most capable person in the world	.615	.437
Consumption (first-order)		
I often use money to buy things related to my idol	.673	.419
I never care about money spent on my idol	.659	.445
I like to buy things related to my idol	.743	.403
Celebrity Attitudes Scale (CAS)		
Entertainment/socializing (first-order)		
My friends and I like to discuss what my favorite celebrity has done	.534	.402
One of the main reasons I maintain an interest in my favorite celebrity is that doing so gives me a temporary escape from life's problems	.591	.414
I enjoy watching, reading, or listening to my favorite celebrity because it means a good time	.651	.417
I love to talk with others who admire my favorite celebrity	.563	.415
When something bad happens to my favorite celebrity I feel like it happened to me	.635	.446
Learning the life story of my favorite celebrity is a lot of fun	.667	.405
It is enjoyable just to be with others who like my favorite celebrity	.660	.416
When my favorite celebrity fails or loses at something I feel like a failure myself	.666	.439
I like watching and hearing about my favorite celebrity when I am in a large group of people	.637	.407
Keeping up with news about my favorite celebrity is an entertaining pastime	.608	.410
Personalizing (intense-personal) (first-order)		
If I were to meet my favorite celebrity in person, he/she would already somehow know that I am his/her biggest fan	.452	.477
I share with my favorite celebrity a special bond that cannot be described in words	.571	.443
I am obsessed by details of my favorite celebrity's life	.662	.423

(*continued*)

Table 3.3 Standardized factor loadings estimated for Model 2 (*continued*)

Factor/indicator	Trait	Method
Factor/indicator		
When something good happens to my favorite celebrity I feel like it happened to me	.658	.412
I have pictures and/or souvenirs of my favorite celebrity which I always keep in exactly the same place	.635	.405
The successes of my favorite celebrity are my successes also	.526	.462
I consider my favorite celebrity to be my soulmate	.589	.440
I have frequent thoughts about my favorite celebrity, even when I don't want to	.759	.399
When my favorite celebrity dies (or died) I will feel (or felt) like dying too	.477	.423
Obsession (pathological) (first-order)		
I often feel compelled to learn the personal habits of my favorite celebrity	.540	.435
If I were lucky enough to meet my favorite celebrity, and he/she asked me to do something illegal as a favor, I would probably do it	.285	.503
If someone gave me several thousand dollars to do with as I please, I would consider spending it on a personal possession (like a napkin or paper plate) once used by my favorite celebrity	.426	.520
News about my favorite celebrity is a pleasant break from a harsh world	.655	.415
Second-order factor		
Idol worship (second-order)		
Identification (first-order)	.635	
Attachment (first-order)	.876	
Romanticization (first-order)	.772	
Idealization (first-order)	.702	
Consumption (first-order)	.770	
Celebrity worship (second-order)		
Entertainment/socializing (first-order)	.956	
Personalizing (intense-personal) (first-order)	.980	
Obsession (pathological) (first-order)	.983	

The findings reported in this chapter demonstrate the expected similarities and dissimilarities between AAI and IEI. The two forms of worship are similar in that they are highly correlated but show common gender differences in that young women are more likely than young men to be celebrity worshippers. The findings indicate a need to refine the measures. For instance, the CAS lacks the identification component (Cheung and Yue 2018) and is thus biased against the emulative role in which idols or celebrities serve as reference role models (Austin et al. 2008; Fraser and Brown 2002) rather than as focuses for entertainment, consumption, idealization, romanticization, or attachment (Cheung and Yue 2018). The factors of celebrity worship had very high interfactor correlations or convergence. Weaker intercorrelations (Houran et al. 2005; Maltby, Day, McCutcheon, Martin, and Cayanus 2004; Reeves et al. 2012) implied that the measures are less suitable to Hong Kong or Western-oriented students (Cheung and Yue 2018).

Summary

AAI and IEI show differences and similarities in idol worship. That is, idol worship can serve purposes beyond evoking fanatic fan club membership, pathological involvement, and fulfillment of entertainment, socializing, personalizing, obsession, and addiction needs. Instead, admirers can use idols as role models for achievement through identification, attachment, romanticization, idealization, and consumption (Lin and Lin 2007). By distinguishing between AAI and IEI, we show that idol worship can be normal and healthy for both older and younger youth in their search for self-identity and protection (Cheng 2017). Secondary school and university students are equally intense in their involvement in celebrity worship (Stevens 2010). Finally, it is encouraging to see that AAI and IEI are largely compatible for measuring the two forms of worship (Cheung and Yue 2018). Specifically, the present measure of AAI has little about identification. This is inadequate as identification with the celebrity as well as the idol is clearly salient. As an idol can very well be a role model, reference, or endorser (Austin et al. 2008; Fraser and Brown 2002), idols or celebrities need not be merely for entertainment, consumption, idealization, romanticization, or attachment; they could also be for aspiration, inspiration, and identification.

4 Idol worship and personality factors

This chapter is a review of studies that have examined how personality factors affect idol worship in Chinese societies.

Idol worship has been associated with parental absence (Cheung and Yue 2012), self-efficacy (Cheung and Yue 2003b), coping styles (Maltby, Day, McCutcheon, Gillett, Houran, and Ashe 2004), and personality traits. A study of 317 British university students and 290 adults revealed that extroverted students are most likely to be involved in the entertainment-social levels of celebrity worship; neurotic students are more likely to be involved in the intense-personal levels of celebrity worship; and pathologically disturbed students are more likely to be involved in the pathological levels of celebrity worship (Eysenck, Eysenck, and Barrett 1985; Maltby, Beriault, Watson, Liepert, and Fick 2003). As measured by the Celebrity Attitude Scale (CAS), the entertainment-social level indicates extroversion traits such as activeness, sociability, and vigor; the intense-personal level indicates neurotic features such as emotionality and tenseness; and the pathological level indicates psychotic features such as egocentrism and impulsivity. Idol worship has been positively correlated with the entertainment-social level as measured by the CAS and with extroversion according to Eysenck's personality theory (Eysenck and Eysenck 1975; Maltby, Houran, and McCutcheon 2003). Conversely, intense-personal worship has been positively correlated with neuroticism; pathological worship has been positively correlated with psychoticism.

In addition to Eysenck's personality model (Eysenck and Eysenck 1975), idol worship studies have used the five-factor model of personality (e.g., Batey, Chamorro-Premuzic, and Furnham 2009; Chappelle, Novy, Sowin, and Thompson 2010). That is, intense-personal worship has been closely associated with neuroticism (Maltby and Day 2001; Maltby, Beriault, Watson, Liepert, and Fick 2003; Maltby, Day, McCutcheon, Gillett, Houran, and Ashe 2004). Entertaining-social worship has been closely associated with extroversion (Maltby, Beriault, Watson, Liepert, and Fick 2003). Intense-personal celebrity worship has been associated with neuroticism, based on the revised NEO personality inventory (NEO PI-R; Maltby, McCutcheon, and Lowinger 2011). Entertaining-social celebrity worship has been associated with extroversion in the NEO PI-R. However, the associations did not include gender differentials.

Self-esteem, self-efficacy, and idol worship

Personality is formed according to how individuals perceive and evaluate themselves. Five-factor model studies argue that self-esteem is positively associated with extroversion and conscientiousness and negatively associated with neuroticism (Goldberg and Rosolack 1994; Pullman and Allik 2000; Robins, Hendin, and Trzesniewski 2001). Cross-cultural studies have found similar results showing that self-esteem is associated with several socially desirable personality traits (Robins, Hendin, and Trzesniewski 2001).

Entertainment-social worship has been significantly and positively related with extroversion (Maltby, Houran, and McCutcheon 2003). Intense-personal worship has been positively correlated with neuroticism. Pathological worship has been correlated with psychoticism. In a study of 329 participants of diverse ages living in Northern England, Maltby, McCutcheon, and Lowinger (2011) found a positive relationship between intense-personal worship and neuroticism. Entertainment-social celebrity worship was also positively related with extroversion.

Individuals who have self-efficacy believe that their efforts will bring success. They have an internal locus of control, meaning that they believe that success or failure depends on internal or controllable factors. In contrast, individuals who have an external locus of control believe that external or uncontrollable factors such as luck and task difficulty determine success or failure (Bandura 1997). Self-perceived self-efficacy and self-consciousness both pertain to social perception. Theoretically, identity confusion causes self-consciousness, while identity achievement generates a positive sense of self-direction, certainty, and self-esteem (Erikson 1968). Similarly, mature identity indicates self-efficacy.

Self-efficacy is closely associated with mature identity, which in turn is associated with moral reasoning, self-esteem, personal autonomy, and internal control (Abraham, Potegal, and Miller 1983; Adams and Shea 1979). High self-efficacy benefits adolescents by contributing to cognitive, motivational, affective, and selection development. Self-efficacy also contributes to academic development by shaping beliefs in abilities to achieve aspirations and academic success (Bandura 1993).

Self-efficacy may be relevant to types of idol worship. Self-efficacy theory argues that individuals construct self-efficacy perceptions through previous successes or failures or through vicarious experiences of others' successes or failures. When individuals observe others experiencing success, they will have rising self-efficacy; when they see others experiencing failure, self-efficacy deteriorates, especially if they regard themselves as similar to the model. If adolescents consider their peers as having similar ability, peer success may increase self-efficacy. Therefore, when idols have achieved success because of uncontrollable external factors such as image, worshippers may perceive that they have no control over their success, thus reducing self-efficacy. Conversely, when role models have achieved success because of controllable internal factors such as talent and moral conduct, admirers may perceive that success comes from mastery, thus raising self-efficacy.

Attachment, self-esteem, loneliness, and idol worship

Lonely people feel "a sense of isolation that persists over time" (Perse and Rubin 1990). They tend to lack communication skills, with consequent detachment from social activities. Uses and gratification theory explains that when individuals cannot satiate their social needs in normal ways, they may turn to idol or celebrity worship to find connections (Rubin, Perse, and Powell 1985), but their relationships will be one-sided and nondemanding (McCutcheon, Aruguete, Scott, and Von Waldner 2004). They can imagine intimacy without the discomfort of ordinary interactions (McCutcheon et al. 2004).

However, loneliness and solitude are both weakly correlated with idol worship (Ashe and McCutcheon 2001; McCutcheon et al. 2004) and would thus be negatively related to celebrity attachment. Men and women who show high intense-personal celebrity worship tend to be high in neuroticism (Maltby, Houran, and McCutcheon 2003; Maltby, McCutcheon, and Lowinger 2011), unable to cope with stress, and more likely to be mentally ill (Maltby, Day, McCutcheon, Gillett, Houran, and Ashe 2004). In contrast, men and women who show high entertainment-social celebrity worship tend to be high in extroversion.

Gender significantly predicts idol selection (Adams-Price and Greene 1990; Teigen, Normann, Bjorkheim, and Helland 2000). In the past, women were more focused on desires for family and romantic relationships and tended to form illusory romantic relationships based on physical appearance, while men generally experienced greater career pressures and were more likely to focus on achievement and internal traits (Adams-Price and Greene 1990; Teigen et al. 2000). However, we have observed increasing ambiguity regarding sex roles in Hong Kong. That is, with the rise of feminism, women are more focused on careers and economic independence and tend to value both external characteristics (idol illusory romance and idol idealism) and internal traits (idol identification and idol relativism; Yue, Wong, and Cheung 2000; Yue and Cheung 2000a, 2000b). Therefore, women look for both romance and achievement and thus tend to seek information and form ego identity from both glamorous stars and prestigious luminaries. Moreover, participants who had high self-esteem maintained positive relationships with secure attachments; those who lacked self-esteem had negative relationships with preoccupied attachments, which is consistent with extant research. However, self-esteem was not associated with dismissive attachments, a finding that does not accord with extant findings.

A new finding is that fearful attachment was negatively correlated with self-esteem. Attachment styles are associated with the formation of self-image and images of others (Ainsworth 1989; Bartholomew and Horowitz 1991; Bowlby 1973). Both secure and dismissive attachment styles can encourage positive self-images, but both preoccupied and fearful attachment styles encourage negative self-image (Bartholomew and Horowitz 1991). Hence, secure and dismissive attachment styles have often been positively correlated with self-esteem (Arbona and Power 2003; Armitage and Harris 2006; Bartholomew and Horowitz 1991; Brennan and Bosson 1998; Brennan and Morris 1997; Bringle and Bagby 1992; Bylsma, Cozzarelli, and Sumer 1997; Collins and Read 1990; Emmanuelle 2009; Feeney and Noller 1990; Gomez and McLaren 2007; Laible, Carlo, and Roesch 2004; McCormick and Kennedy 1994; Mikulincer 1995, 1998; O'Koon 1997; Ooi, Ang, Fung, Wong, and Cai 2006; Paterson, Pryor, and Field 1995; Wearden, Peters, Berry, Barrowdough, and Liversidge 2008; Wilkinson 2004). Conversely, both fearful and preoccupied attachment styles have been negatively associated with self-esteem (Foster, Kernis, and Goldman 2007; Srivastava and Beer 2005; Wu 2009). However, we found dismissive attachment to be associated with self-esteem, perhaps because attachment styles overlapped with self-esteem to affect self-perceived competence. Attachment involved interpersonal interaction, a marker of self-worth (Bylsma et al. 1997).

Thus, idol worshippers are likely to feel more positive about themselves when they receive positive feedback from other fans and when they talk about their shared admiration for idols. However, self-perceived competence involves more than socialization; it requires intrapersonal skills such as academic performance. Since idol worship negatively affects academic achievement (Schultze et al. 1991), we could expect idol worship to have a reversed effect on self-perceived competence. Therefore, idol worship may mediate the relationship between dismissive attachment and self-esteem, but dismissive attachment would be negatively associated with self-esteem. Those predictions arise from our research, so further research is required. In addition, consistent with previous findings, self-esteem was negatively correlated with idol identification, illusory romance, idealism, and prestige orientation.

Preoccupied and dismissive attachment were positively related to social loneliness and emotional loneliness, a new finding. Limited social networks cause social isolation and social loneliness; the lack of intimate relationships generates emotional loneliness (Weiss 1973). Securely attached individuals are likely to have positive views of themselves and others and will be able to establish satisfying social networks and intimate relationships with significant others. However, insecurely attached individuals will have deficient intimate relationships. Numerous studies have consistently shown that loneliness is positively associated with secure attachment and negatively associated with insecure attachment (Bartholomew 1990; DiTommaso, Brannen-McNulty, Ross, and Burgess 2003; Larose, Guay, and Boivin 2002; Wiseman, Mayseless, and Sharabany 2006). Loneliness was not significantly correlated with any dimension of idol worship, which contradicts previous findings that loneliness was weakly associated with idol worship (Ashe and McCutcheon 2001). However, the insignificant findings are reasonable considering the weak correlations found in extant studies.

Among four attachment styles, preoccupied attachment was found to be significantly and positively correlated with idol identification, idol illusory romance, idol relativism, idol worship expense, opposite-sex attraction, prestige orientation, and glamour orientation (Cheng 2017). As individuals transition to adulthood, idol worship marks the second attachment in the attempt to acquire a secure base through an imaginative relationship with an idol. Preoccupied individuals view themselves negatively but view others positively, have low self-confidence, and feel unworthy (Bartholomew and Horowitz 1991), but they indicated intense reliance and romantic feelings toward a significant idol, particularly coaches. A particular feature of preoccupied attachment is that individuals are more likely to idealize and rely on others (Bartholomew and Horowitz 1991). They particularly need security; thus, idol worship is a way to refine their interests and values while exercising their scripts regarding intimacy (Job 2002; Lerner and Olson 1995). In addition, their self-diffidence causes them to idolize the opposite sex and to fear rejection (Job 2002; Lerner and Olson 1995). Preoccupied attachment was also strongly and positively associated with idol worship.

Fearful attachment indicates a lack of self-confidence, particularly in self-expression. Individuals who have fearful attachment are generally less likely to be involved in intimate relationships because they fear rejection and thus avoid the actual pursuit of love. They are likely to show idol illusory romance, opposite-sex attraction, achievement orientation, prestige orientation, glamour orientation, and concern about romantic relationships. The strong desire for intimate relationships then shifts to the desire for idols located at safe distances. Therefore, fearful attachment would be modestly related with idol worship.

Cheng (2017) examined 791 students regarding self-esteem, four attachment styles, and rejection sensitivity according to those who showed the lowest (30%), the middle (40%), and the highest (30%) levels of fandom (Table 4.1). The study showed no significant level differences in self-esteem ($F(2,654) = 1.215$, $p = .297$), rejection sensitivity ($F(2,654) = 0.81$, $p = .445$), and preoccupied attachment ($F(2,654) = 0.898$, $p = .408$). By contrast, the levels showed significant differences

Table 4.1 Attachment styles, self-esteem, and rejection sensitivity for levels of fandom

				Fandom measure (N = 657)		
Variable		F(2,654)	p	Lowest 30% (n = 192)	Middle 40% (n = 268)	Highest 30% (n = 197)
Attachment styles	Preoccupied attachment style	0.898	.408			
	M±SD			4.71±1.05	4.58±1.06	4.62±0.99
	Dismissive attachment style	4.505	.011			
	M±SD			4.31±0.98	4.32±0.83	4.08±0.91
	Fearful attachment style	2.986	.051			
	M±SD			3.87±1.05	3.72±0.92	3.63±0.99
	Secure attachment style	2.525	.081			
	M±SD			4.08±0.81	4.18±0.81	4.26±0.81
Self-esteem	Self-esteem	1.215	.297			
	M±SD			27.95±5.36	28.56±5.36	28.76±5.32
Rejection sensitivity	Rejection sensitivity	0.81	.445			
	M±SD			10.14±3.84	9.82±3.59	9.68±3.40

in secure attachment ($F(2,654) = 2.525$, $p = .081$), fearful attachment, ($F(2,654) = 2.986$, $p = .051$), and dismissive attachment ($F(2,654) = 4.505$, $p = .011$).

The highest level of the fandom measure showed significantly lower dismissive attachment (4.08 ± 0.91) than did the middle (4.32 ± 0.83, $p = .014$) and lowest levels (4.31 ± 0.98, $p = .006$). Furthermore, the highest level had significantly lower fearful attachment (3.63 ± 0.99) than did the lowest 30% (3.87 ± 1.05, $p = .016$) and significantly higher secure attachment (4.26 ± 0.81) than did the lowest 30% (4.08 ± 0.81, $p = .025$). The dismissive attachment of the highest level of fandom was significantly lower than the middle and lowest levels. Moreover, the fearful attachment of the highest level of fandom was significantly lower than that of the lowest level and showed no difference from that of the middle level. Secure attachment at the highest level of fandom was significantly higher than that of the lowest level and showed no difference from that of the middle level. Self-esteem, rejection sensitivity, and preoccupied attachment showed no significant differences among the three levels of fandom.

The results indicate that fandom is psychologically normal rather than pathological. Moreover, serious fandom was associated with healthy psychosocial conditions. Essentially, the fandom measure appeared reliable.

Summary

The foregoing paragraphs discussed studies conducted in Hong Kong that examined how idol worship was related to attachment styles, loneliness, self-esteem, self-efficacy, and so on. There appears to be a general tendency that strong idol worshippers, particularly adolescents, were likely to be lonely and insecurely attached and to have low self-esteem during adolescence. This finding needs to be verified in future studies using both experimental and longitudinal research designs. Further research is also needed to measure the influence of star idols that is immune to the individual's self-selection (i.e., even though worship of idols or star idols may not be the root cause of retarded youth development, it may function as an important mediator that reinforces the effect of the root cause). The longitudinal design of further research should be able to clarify how idol worship plays a mediating and even moderating role that may amplify the effect of the root cause. In addition, analysis of star idols' images, performances, products, and dispositional characteristics is also recommended to determine how worship of star idols may result in developmental problems for adolescents. Earlier studies tend to project star idols as being repetitive and uncreative, having a hedonistic and luxurious lifestyle, and conveying cynical, antisocial, vulgar, unintelligible, and unintelligent messages (Greeson and Williams 1986; Lull 1987; Schultze et al. 1991). Mass media in Hong Kong also reveal that many pop stars are unknowledgeable and unscrupulous in their everyday life. Nevertheless, it is ironic that these uncultured manners appear to be highly attractive to their young fans. Further research should conduct adequate quantitative content analysis and qualitative discourse and hermeneutic analysis of pop stars and their sponsors to unravel the causal root.

5 Religiosity, self-identity, and idol worship

Idol worship and religious orientation

Religiosity is highly connected with idol worship (Maltby, Houran, Lange, Ashe, and McCutcheon 2002). Religious orientation indicates a "general disposition to use particular means to attain particular ends in living" (Pargament 1997). *Religiosity* has been defined in terms of three distinctive religious orientations: (1) *intrinsic orientation*, involving full commitment to religious beliefs, (2) *extrinsic orientation*, involving the use of religion for social gain, and (3) *quest*, concerning the open-ended search for answers to existential, paradoxical, and uncertain questions (Allport 1950; Batson, Scheonrade, and Ventis 1993).

Attachment theory explains how individuals form an attachment to a Supreme Being (Bowlby 1969). Attachment is an affectionate bond with a figure serving both as a secure base for exploring and a refuge for comfort and security (Ainsworth 1985). Attachment styles appear to be similar to religious beliefs, particularly Christian beliefs (Kirkpatrick 1999). Accordingly, personal attachment becomes focused on God (Granqvist 1998; Kirkpatrick 1997, 1999). Attachment to God can be viewed in terms of *anxiety about abandonment* and *avoidance of intimacy* (Beck and McDonald 2004). Worshippers who have anxiety about abandonment worry about their relationship with God and fear that God will abandon them. In contrast, worshippers who tend to avoid intimacy desire to be self-reliant and independent and are reluctant to maintain an emotional connection with God. Researchers have not directly investigated the relationship between religious orientation and attachment to God (Miner 2009), but a quest orientation has been negatively correlated with an insecure attachment to God (Beck 2006). Attachment to God has been shown to indicate positive attachments to adults, such as parents, and to increase mental health (Kirkpatrick and Shaver 1990, 1992).

One of the Christian Ten Commandments warns against worshipping gods other than the Christian God. Many Christians consider it sinful to worship media stars or luminaries. Indeed, researchers have found that religiosity is negatively associated with idol worship (Giles 2000; Maltby et al. 2002).

Man-tsz Ho (2013) surveyed 220 secondary school students in Hong Kong in an effort to relate idol worship to religiosity and mental health. Students completed the 26-item Idol Worship Questionnaire (IWQ; Yue and Cheung 2000a, 2000b) and the 23-item Celebrity Attitude Scale (CAS). The study focused on the *identification, romantic fantasy*, and *idealization* components of IWQ. Each component included three items, measured on a five-point Likert scale (1 = *strongly disagree* and 5 = *strongly agree*). CAS included *entertainment-social, intense-personal*, and *pathological* levels and measured worship on a five-point Likert scale (1 = *strongly disagree* and 5 = *strongly agree*).

Participants also completed the ten-item Rosenberg Self-Esteem Scale, a unidimensional scale designed to measure global self-esteem (Rosenberg 1965) on a four-point Likert scale (1 = *strongly disagree* and 4 = *strongly agree*). They also completed the four-item Subjective Happiness Scale, a measure of global subjective happiness. The scale consists of four items rated on a seven-point scale (1 = *very unhappy* and 7 = *very happy*). It maintained good reliability (Cronbach's α = .86; Lyubomirsky and Lepper 1999).

Finally, participants completed three scales measuring religious attachment and religious orientation: the 28-item Attachment to God Inventory (AGI), the 12-item Quest Scale, and the 12-item Age Universal I-E Scale (AUIE). AGI assessed two dimensions of attachment to God: *anxiety about abandonment* and *avoidance of intimacy*. Each dimension included 14 items answered on a seven-point Likert scale (1 = *strongly disagree* and 7 = *strongly agree*). The Quest Scale measured quest orientation toward religion (Batson and Scheonrade 1991a, 1991b), including three factors: *complexity, doubt*, and *tentativeness*. Each subscale had four items, all measured on a three-point scale (1 = *no*, 2 = *not certain*, 3 = *yes*). AUIE is an amendment of the Religious Orientation Scale (Allport and Ross 1967), the most renowned measure of intrinsic and extrinsic religious orientations. Essentially, AUIE condenses the original 20 items into 12 items to attain higher reliability and validity than the original scale (Maltby 1999; Maltby et al. 2002). It comprises three subscales: *intrinsic* (six items), *extrinsic-personal* (three items), and *extrinsic-social* (three items), measured on a three-point scale (1 = *no*, 2 = *not certain*, 3 = *yes*).

Young women scored higher than young men on IWQ and CAS. Significant differences appeared in the romantic fantasy, entertainment-social, and intense-personal dimensions of worship. The findings echo previous findings that women have more romantic fantasies and illusions about their favored idols than do men (Adams-Price and Greene 1990; Cheung and Yue 2000, 2003a, 2003b; Yue and Cheung 2000a, 2000b). The higher entertainment-social dimension of idol worship among young women may reflect their higher social cohesion (Yue and Yan 2009). Moreover, fan club members scored significantly higher than nonmembers on CAS, except at pathological levels, consistent with previous findings that fan club members are significantly more committed to idolatry (e.g., Cheung and Yue 2003a, 2003b). Christians generally scored higher than non-Christians on religiosity scales. The pathological and entertainment-social levels of worship significantly predicted a lack of attachment to God.

Idol worship and self-identity

Identity indicates how individuals define themselves according to their internal beliefs. In late adolescence, individuals develop their perceptions of their judgment and efficacy skills (Marcia 1993). Theoretically, identity formation is a process of personal exploration leading to a coherent set of attitudes, values, and beliefs (Erikson 1963). Marcia (1993) conceptualized identity development based on whether individuals have considered diverse options and have become committed to a vocation, religion, sexual orientation, and political stance.

Identity has four status conditions: identity diffusion, foreclosure, moratorium, and achievement. Adolescents who have identity diffusion lack the ability to explore and commit. They have failed to find an occupational direction or an ideological commitment and show little progress in doing so. If and when they experience an identity crisis, they may be unable to resolve it. Foreclosure occurs when adolescents have commitment but lack adequate exploration. Rather than experiencing an identity crisis, they adopt identities prematurely according to their parents' choices rather than their own. They show occupational and ideological commitments, but the commitments reflect the preference of parents or other authority figures. The result is a pseudo-identity that is too inflexible to meet the demands of future life crises. Moratorium adolescents lack firm commitment and are actively exploring their occupational and ideological choices without commitment. Such adolescents are experiencing identity crises. They will achieve identity only after personal exploration and autonomous, genuine, voluntary commitment.

In contrast to the other adolescents in the study, Hong Kong moratorium adolescents were more likely to learn from role models (Lin and Lin 2007). Foreclosed adolescents were more likely to worship idols, perhaps because they scored lower on cognitive ability, notably critical thinking and creativity (McCutcheon, Ashe, Houran, and Maltby 2003), and tended to be less analytical or philosophical (Read, Adams, and Dobson 1984). Unsurprisingly, moratorium adolescents were more likely to learn adaptive social skills from role models, whereas foreclosed adolescents were less likely to learn adaptive social skills. Star idol fans were shown to have low self-esteem; in contrast, admirers of luminaries scored higher on perceived self-efficacy (Cheng 1997; Cheung and Yue 2003a, 2003b).

Moreover, moratorium adolescents scored higher on all dimensions of the IWQ, indicating that moratorium adolescents identify with their idols (see Figure 5.1). They indicated having lower satisfaction with their situation because they experienced higher social pressure (Waterman and Waterman 1972). To achieve self-identity, they tended to model their behavior after their idols, in contrast to their foreclosed counterparts, perhaps because model learning focuses on the model's ability and achievement. Thus, they learned social and cognitive maturity from the model. Uncommitted adolescents, compared to committed adolescents, paid more attention to social information and were more deeply concerned about their social environment (Adams, Ryan, Hoffman, Dobson, and Nielsen 1985).

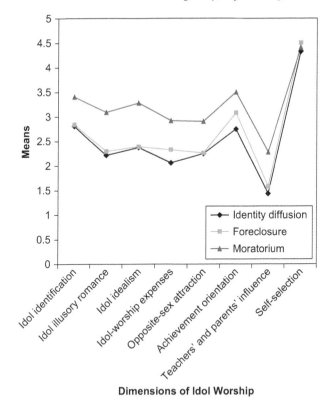

Figure 5.1 Ego identity status patterns in different dimensions of idol worship

By contrast, idol worship is extremely based on *idealism-romanticism-absolutism* and focused on the idols' external traits, fulfilling illusory romance and vainglory desires.

Cheung and Yue (2003b) conducted a computer-assisted telephone survey of a random sample of 833 Hong Kong teenagers about the relationship between idol worship, identity achievement, and self-esteem. Identity achievement was found to be susceptible to the negative influence of exposure to star idols, resulting in illusory romance, reification, vainglory, fan-club membership, and years of idol worship. Virtually all factors related to idol worship led to poorer identity achievement. These findings clearly reveal aversive effects of idol worship as a way to promote identity achievement. The effects may stem from illusory romance, reification, and vainglory, which may reflect materialism, commodity fetishism, and irrationality (Leonard 1984; Sherlock 1997). These orientations may alienate the teenager from being conscious about the self and the collective. As a result, the teenager has little exposure, exploration, and commitment to family, work, religion, and political thought and activities. In addition, worship of a nonstar was found to be detrimental to the identity achievement of teenagers who are not star fans. It is likely that worship of a nonstar involves the same alienating mechanism as worship of a star to cut the teenager off from the self and collective. Behavioral and attitudinal indulgence in the worship of both star and nonstar idols therefore does not seem to foster the teenager's identity achievement.

On the other hand, identification also predicts idol worship. Children and adolescents commonly see specific celebrities as their heroes (Giles and Maltby 2004). By identifying with adult idols, developing children and adolescents acquire information about the values associated with adult roles (Erikson 1968). They identify with the manners and values associated with the idol, and thus the idol becomes a role model for attaining identity.

Strong ego identity indicates self-acceptance and direction; weak ego identity indicates self-doubt and inability to make decisions or commitments. Theoretically, strong ego identity gives stability and integrity (Erikson 1950). The absorption-addiction model explains that individuals may become absorbed in celebrity worship to forge an identity and find fulfillment (McCutcheon, Lange, and Houran 2002). Consequently, extreme celebrity worship may indicate deficient ego identity. Identity achievement and self-esteem are essential for adolescents to avoid worry and preoccupation, depression, diffusion, and aimlessness. Model learning is a way for adolescents to achieve identity (Erikson 1968).

The worship of star idols appears to be harmful to adolescent development. For example, fans who adore heavy-metal singers tend to show misbehavior such as sexual promiscuity and drug addiction (Martin and Segrave 1988). The worship of star idols tends to encourage vainglory and illusory romance (Arnett 1991; Wan 1997). Intense celebrity worship has been associated with psychopathology, fantasy, and dissociation, while intense-personal and borderline-pathological celebrity worship has been negatively related with ego identity (Maltby, Day, McCutcheon, Houran, and Ashe 2006).

In contrast, rather than harm adolescent development, the worship of luminary idols appears to motivate adolescents to pursue their goals. Hence, students can form their identities and develop aspirations for the future by modeling the behavior of celebrity figures (Yue and Cheung 2000a, 2000b). Social learning theory explains that people can modify their behavior by observing social punishments or rewards for behaviors (Bandura 1986). In support, a study showed that students who were in a group that observed a model performing motor skills learned better than students in a control group receiving minimal verbal instructions (Hayes, Ashford, and Bennett 2008). Thus, observational learning from a model shows observers specific imitative ways to attain goals. Consequently, we suggest that if the success of idols was demystified, adolescents might gain more benefits from idol worship (Yue, Cheung, and Wong 2010; Cheung and Yue 2018).

Lam (2013) surveyed 244 adult fan-club members using the IWQ, the CAS, the Attachment Style Questionnaire, and the Rosenberg Self-Esteem Scale. Results showed idolatrous behaviors sustained into adulthood, and female club members scored significantly higher than their male counterparts on

Table 5.1 Gender differences in idol worship

| | Males (n = 62) | | Females (n = 175) | | |
	M	SD	M	SD	t
Idol Worship Questionnaire					
Emotional attachment	17.44	5.86	19.62	5.50	−2.64**
Idol selection criteria	16.08	3.65	15.95	4.23	.21
Inspiration and personal projection	16.60	5.15	16.65	5.39	−.06
Worship influence	5.61	2.23	5.29	2.40	.94
Romantic fantasy	10.00	4.28	11.90	4.59	−2.85**
Celebrity Attitude Scale					
Entertainment-social	28.68	8.91	31.97	8.18	−2.66**
Intense-personal	22.03	7.27	24.75	7.66	−2.43*
Borderline-pathological	8.55	3.11	8.35	2.99	.45

Notes
*$p < .05$
**$p < .1$

the emotional-attachment and romantic-fantasy dimensions of IWQ and the entertainment-social and intense-personal dimensions of CAS (Table 5.1).

To determine further the relative contribution of the combined predictive power, a five-multiple stepwise regression was calculated (Table 5.2). The results for emotional attachment, inspiration and personal projection, idolatrous influence, and

Table 5.2 Multiple-regression analysis on predicting nonpathological idol worship

		ΔR^2	B	SE	β
Entertainment-social					
Step 1		.49***			
	Emotional attachment		1.05***	.07	0.70
Step 5	Emotional attachment	.12***			
	Inspiration and personal projection		.76***	.07	.50
	Preoccupation with relationship		.18***	.06	.13
	Worship influence		.38**	.16	.11
	Idol selection criteria		.22**	.10	.10
Intense-personal					
Step 1		.52***			
	Emotional attachment		.99***	.06	.72
Step 5		.13***			
	Emotional attachment		.65***	.07	.48
	Inspiration and personal projection		.21*	.08	.15
	Preoccupation with relationship		.14**	.05	.11
	Worship influence		.61***	.14	.19
	Romantic fantasy		.26*	.10	.16

Notes
*$p <. 05$
**$p < .01$
***$p < .001$

idol selection were all statistically significant and predicted an entertainment-social level of idol worship under the CAS, $F(5,231) = 72.10$, $p < .001$, adj. $R^2 = .60$. The model was also statistically significant and predicted an intense-personal level of idol worship, $F(5,231) = 83.48$, $p < .001$, adj. $R^2 = .64$.

Ho (2008) examined the relationships among parental styles, idol worship, and self-efficacy among a sample of 205 students (106 high school students and 99 university students) in Hong Kong. The results showed that students with permissive fathers tended to be more engaged in romantic fantasy and idealism toward their admired idols, whereas students with permissive mothers tended to have more self-efficacy than those with undifferentiated and authoritarian mothers. In addition, students with permissive mothers also idolized star idols more than those with authoritative mothers. Taken together, students with permissive parents appear to identify with and idealize their idols more than their counterparts with authoritarian parents. Students may identify with and idealize idols if their parents are unable to mediate their building of personal identity (Lapsley, Rice, and Fitzgerald 1990). Therefore, it is no surprise that in the present study, parental authoritativeness was negatively correlated with idol worship, and parental authoritarianism was positively correlated with idol worship.

Summary

Identity achievement involves exploration of and eventually commitment to goals about one's career, sexuality and marriage, family, religion and beliefs, community, and political involvement (Erikson 1968; Kroger 1996). According to past research and theory, identity achievement tends to result from holding critical views toward parents and societal issues, being autonomous and independent from the family, and actively participating in school (Adams, Ryan & Keating 2000; Kamptner 1988; Waterman and Archer 1993). Close relationships with parents and family cohesion tend to foster identity foreclosure, which predisposes the youngster to premature conformity to expectations of authority figures (Marcia 1980). The research findings above suggest that worship of parents and family members may not necessarily contribute to the teenager's identity achievement. They instead indicate that being critical and nonconforming to parental dictates may pave the road to the teenager's identity achievement. Therefore, worship of star idols and nonstar idols alike would not nourish identity achievement. Interesting as these findings may appear, studies on the relationship between idolatrous behaviors and religiosity as well as dispositional factors are rare and sporadic in Chinese societies. Previous studies generally show that worship of star idols appears to be harmful to adolescent development, whereas worship of luminary idols appears to motivate adolescents to pursue their goals. Adolescents can form their identities and develop aspirations for the future by modeling the behavior of celebrity figures. As such, parents and schoolteachers ought to take a more accommodating view of the potential facilitating role of idol worship on adolescents' identity formation and self-development. More studies, experimental or otherwise, ought to be conducted to identify and verify such positive connections (Yue et al. 2010).

6 Idolatry, self-efficacy, attachment, and intimacy

Part 1: Existing possibilities

Elucidating *idolatry* in relation to *self-efficacy* belief, *attachment*, and *intimacy* is necessary to refine one's understanding about idolatry. In brief, *idolatry* or *idol worship* refers to an attitude or practice highly in favor of an idol, which means a figure that is highly instructive and/or venerable (McCutcheon, Lange, and Houran 2002). *Self-efficacy* belief means belief in one's generalized efficacy in tackling problems or achieving goals (Schwarzer, Mueller, and Greenglass 1999). It is thus a favorable attitude toward oneself. *Attachment* refers to a positive feeling in relation to people who are significant in one's life (Cotterell 2007). *Intimacy* refers to a close positive relationship with a person (Christopher, Poulsen, and McKenney 2016). Attachment is most general, as it applies to any other people, and self-efficacy belief, intimacy, and idolatry are less general, as they apply to a specific person or figure. Despite the generality or specificity, idolatry, self-efficacy belief, attachment, and intimacy share the common reference of a positive relationship with one self or others. Moreover, idolatry is likely to maintain a positive relationship or spillover with self-efficacy belief, attachment, and intimacy due to an integrated theoretical framework based on attachment theory and symbolic consistency theory (Cole and Leets 1999; Henderson, Hayslip, Sanders, and Louden 2009). Contrariwise, negative relationships or compensation between idolatry and other engagements are plausible, according to the compensation thesis (Argyle 1994; Feldman and Wentzel 1995; Jenson 1992). In any case, such relationships are particularly relevant to youth, to whom idolatry, self-efficacy belief, attachment, and intimacy are prominent (Bendicksen 2013; Cote 2014). Clarifying the relationships is an essential task for review and scrutiny.

Idolatry comprises idolizing of idols, choosing idols, and accepting them as idols or models. Accordingly, idolatry encompasses different ways of idolizing different kinds of idols. *Idolizing* herein refers to the way of relating to or worshipping an idol. Based on a functionalist conceptualization, the 11 primary ways of idolizing are *idealizing, beautifying, crediting, glamourizing, modeling, commodifying, framing, romanticizing, befriending, popularizing,* and *personalizing.* Specifically, idealizing, beautifying, crediting, glamourizing, and modeling represent the primary function of fulfillment or goal attainment. Commodifying and faming serve the primary function of adaptation. Romanticizing, befriending, and popularizing uphold the primary function of integration. Lastly, personalizing reflects the primary function of latency or pattern maintenance. Moreover, beautifying and romanticizing endorse the fulfillment function at the secondary level. Crediting, commodifying, and befriending buttress the adaptation function at the secondary level. Glamourizing, faming, and popularizing sustain the integration function at the secondary level. Finally, modeling and personalizing champion the latency function at the secondary level. Such idolizing applies to at least 30 ways of classifying idols, namely, the Western, Japanese, female (vs. male), entertainment, athletic, academic, ideological, literary, political, military, business, historical, fictional, familial, parent, teacher, peer, heroic, altruistic, idealistic, scientist, musical, mathematics, professional, artistic, navigating, criminal, star, luminary, and celebrity (vs. noncelebrity) idol. The idol can vary in acceptance as an idol or model, which means a figure of learning or emulation.

Functions of idolizing

In the first place, the functionalist conceptualization of idolizing refers to regarding idolizing as contributing to the survival or functioning of the person, society, and/or their practice, including idolatry. For instance, the functionalist appeal means that the various forms of idolizing are integral to the operation, manifestation, or definition of idolatry. Typically, the functionalist differentiates four required functions, namely, goal attainment or fulfilling, adaptation, integration, and latency or pattern maintenance (Munch 1987; Parsons 1968). These four functions arise from the crossing of two dimensions of concern, pertaining to an external versus internal dimension and a consummatory versus instrumental dimension. External concerns or resources require the functions of fulfilling and adaptation, whereas internal concerns or resources require the functions of integration and latency. Furthermore, consummatory concerns require the functions of fulfilling and integration, whereas instrumental concerns require the functions of adaptation and latency. *Consummatory concern* means something valuable in itself, whereas *instrumental concern* means something useful for satisfying consummatory concern. That is, fulfillment and integration are intrinsically satisfying, whereas adaptation and latency are satisfying indirectly, through achievement of benefit and value, respectively. As such, fulfillment or goal attainment means realizing talents or strengths, using power or energy, and acting according to the plan or design. Hence, a person good at singing would worship a good singer. *Adaptation* means optimizing gains, which are benefits minus costs based on rationality, calculation, and need. Thus, a person in need of something obtainable from an idol would worship that idol. *Integration* means conforming to norms or other people through learning and reception of social influence. Thus, a person would worship a popular idol. *Latency* means maintaining consistency with one's beliefs, values, or other ideas in terms of symbolization and enculturation. In this regard, a person would worship an agreeable idol.

Table 6.1 Functionalist conceptualization of idolizing

Primary function	Generic	Secondary function			
		Fulfillment	*Adaptation*	*Integration*	*Latency*
Fulfillment	Idealizing *Glorifying*	Beautifying	Crediting	Glamourizing	Modeling
Adaptation	*Prizing*		Commodifying	Faming	
Integration		Romanticizing	Befriending	Popularizing	
Latency					Personalizing

The *functionalist conceptualization* has the elegant flexibility of functional sectorization (Turner 1986). Accordingly, functions can unfold hierarchically, including primary, secondary, and other subordinate functions. This means that the primary function of fulfillment can encompass the secondary functions of fulfillment, adaptation, integration, and latency. In other words, this is the feature of a fractal, which means something maintaining the same structure even in different scales. This feature allows for the proliferation of subtypes by nesting functions hierarchically. These types or subtypes, to be functionalist, would be functional, satisfying, or fulfilling of functional requirements. Regarding idolatry, idolizing divides into the following 11 primary forms (see Table 6.1).

Idealizing means extolling the idol as an ideal figure, being superlative, insuperable, and the best (Greenwood 2007; Kappes, Schwörer, and Oettingen 2012; Reysen, Plante, Roberts, and Gerbasi 2016). In other words, idealizing holds an idol as an ideal to emulate (Table 6.2). Such an idol figure would meet

Table 6.2 Idolizing

Idolizing	Idol quality	Idol worship
Glamourizing	Glamour	Indulging
Beautifying	Attractiveness	Adoring
		Appreciating
Faming	Fame	Honoring
		Acclaiming
Crediting	Success	Admiring
	Talent	Esteeming
Commodifying	Commodity	Purchasing
		Objectifying
Idealizing	Ideal	Courting
Befriending	Friend	Befriending
	Warmth	Attachment
Romanticizing	Romance	Loving
Personalizing	Fit	Cherishing
Modeling	Model	Learning
		Emulation
		Identifying
Popularizing	Popularity	Conforming
Glorifying	Glory	Following
Prizing	Value	Prizing

the fulfillment function of realizing the talent or ideal through projection onto the idol. Accordingly, the idol would be an ideal human, animal, or another species for fulfilling a corresponding ideal. This setting of an ideal or idealization reflects the need for perfection, which means realizing talents, strengths, or achievements. Such a need is functional to or characteristic of hope, maintenance of pleasure, and defense against failure (Fein 1999). Accordingly, setting an ideal fulfills the need for hope and success. Idealization is also a natural manifestation of emotion in the person and maintenance in society (Bunge 1996; Fein 1999). That is, the person has an ideal about what is good in the persona and society. In the moral or ethical aspect, the ideal is to show the person's rationality and ability to universalize something that is good for all people (Bronuer 2002; Gamble 2010). The ideal can also take other characteristics, including being wealthy, beautiful, intelligent, critical, dutiful, tender, efficient, knowledgeable, fair, tolerant, purposive, religious, and valuable (Bronuer 2002; Bunge 1996; Fein 1999; Gamble 2010). Essential in such idealization are the perspectives of pluralism, feminism, and critical ideology. According to pluralism, the ideal needs to be open, knowledgeable, broadminded, tolerant, and sociable in order to realize the talent to get along well with others or society. Feminism, by contrast, upholds an ideal to be warm, nurturing, amiable, and specifically mothering. With critical ideology, the ideal needs to be intelligent, crucial, fair, reflective, and communicative. In all, the ideal is a referent for ability and/or performance (Bronuer 2002). For instance, one aspiring to achieve academically would idealize an idol for reference to fulfill the aspiration. Idealization is an attempt to connect to the idol.

In achieving the *fulfillment function*, idealization generally appears to be functional, instrumental, satisfying, or salutary. Specifically, idealization of romance or the romantic partner tends to sustain romantic quality (Niehuis 2006). Idealization of the partner or romantic relation is also a prerequisite for dating (Cavanagh 2007; Farrer and Gavin 2009). Similarly, idealization of marriage or the spouse is essential to marriage or its valuation (Bonds-Raacke, Bearden, Carriere, Anderson, and Nicks 2001). In the same vein, sexual idealization can buttress the sexual relationship (Cavanagh 2007). Moreover, idealization is helpful in sustaining prosocial behavior (Csikai and Rosensky 1997), and ethical idealization prevents support for violence (Marcotte 2016). Nevertheless, idealization facilitates learning, even about violent behavior (Greenwood 2007). In addition, idealization helps consolidate attitude (Klaczynski et al. 2009). Idealization such as regarding a figure as omnipotent is a characteristic of youth, specifically of adolescence (Bendicksen 2013). Accordingly, youths need to idealize someone in order to navigate this critical developmental time.

Beautifying means regarding the idol as a beautiful woman, as a handsome man, or as someone who is physically attractive and worthy of adoring or appreciating (Alexander 2010; Boon and Lomore 2001; Rusch et al. 2015). In terms of the functionalist perspective, beautifying serves the primary and secondary functions of fulfillment in realizing physical strength or attractiveness. Both functions concern fulfillment because they reflect a physical or natural property rather than a sensual, social, or ideological property. As such, beautifying represents a projection of one's desire for a physical look similar to the idol's. Hence, a beautiful person is likely to beautify his or her idol (Sivami et al. 2010). Beauty and attractiveness are important in that they signify goodness (Haas and Gregory 2005). Beautifying of the idol thus leads to deference and susceptibility to the idol (Haas and Gregory 2005).

As a functional means, beautifying appears to be instrumental and salutary. Obviously, beautifying of oneself is conducive to self-esteem (Roeser et al. 2008). Beautifying or finding something physically attractive simplifies information processing and thus expedites acceptance (Gambrill 2005). This is attributable to the halo effect generated by beautifying (Montepase and Zebrowitz 2002). This effect facilitates the formation of attitudes and thus judgments. Notably, acceptance of a physically attractive mate is common to facilitate mating (Gangestad et al. 2006). Beautifying of the partner is similarly relevant to romance (Eggermant 2004). Furthermore, beautifying the mentor also raises the effectiveness of mentoring (Johnson et al. 2007). Broadly speaking, beautifying is conducive to relationship building (McCarthy and Casey 2008). More generally, beautifying simulates interest, aspiration, and acquisitiveness (Sheldon and McGregor 2000). Beautifying of an idol particularly enhances investment in the idol (Boon and Lomore 2001). Thus, beautifying plays a motivating function. Moreover, beautifying serves a self-affirmation function to uphold one's self-image, as the beautiful person tends to beautify the idol (Sivami et al. 2010). Beautifying of other people or appreciating their beauty also directly contributes to well-being (Shimai et al. 2006). At the same time, beautifying of oneself makes one confident and facilitates individuation (Hoffman 2014).

Crediting means acclaiming the idol's success, talent, and/or other good features for admiring or esteeming. Thus, crediting or attributing credit to an idol represents admiring the idol (Allison and Goethals 2016; Niu and Wang 2009; Sarapin et al. 2015; Schindler et al. 2013). Furthermore, admiration reflects devotion to the idol (Niu and Wang 2009). Crediting or admiring the idol typically involves the idol's treasurable skill and morality (Sarapin et al. 2015). More generally, the idol's ability is the focus for crediting or admiring. Furthermore, crediting or admiring entails aspiring, observing, learning, emulating, interacting, internalizing, striving, and even belonging to the idol (Schindler et al. 2013). That is, crediting or admiring provides stimulation or energizing (Allison and Goethals 2016). Such stimulation or energizing stems from the motivation to emulate the admired idol (Schindler et al. 2013). Crediting or admiration characterizes idolizing of heroes (Allison and Goethals 2016). Moreover, the admired idol tends to be the prototype of the ideal (Onu et al. 2016).

Crediting or admiring an idol demonstrates fulfillment and adaptation functions in sustaining a good life or performance. Specifically, admiration tends to be generative of prosocial behavior (Algoe and Haidt 2009). Admiration, particularly in the political aspect, is conducive to political participation (Sweetman et al. 2013). Admiration reflects the legitimation of political involvement.

Similarly, admiration of victims instigates unconventional political participation, conceivably in support of the victims (Sweetman et al. 2013). Importantly, admiration also contributes to well-being (van de Ven et al. 2011). Moreover, admiration appears to be motivational, particularly for learning or emulation, or its aspiration or support (Onu et al. 2016; Schindler et al. 2015; van de Ven 2017). Admiration also leads to other forms of commitment, such as affiliation and purchase (Aaker et al. 2012; van de Ven 2017). Conversely, admiration discourages demeaning (van de Ven 2017). In all, admiration sustains personal and social well-being, which includes social integration and cohesion. Hence, admiration is functional to society as well as to the person. This is consistent with the notion that admiration or creating is integral to collectivism, which prizes social well-being (Zemba and Young 2012).

Glamourizing treats the idol as charming and thus induces indulgence (Maltby et al. 2008). It meets the primary function of fulfillment and the secondary function of integration. Accordingly, it fulfills the desire for glamour and integrates people around the glamourized idol. That is, the glamourized idol is enchanting and gathers followers. This indicates that glamour is a basis for popularity (Hakim 2010). Glamourized idols particularly characterize those found in the mass media (Kirsh 2010).

Glamourizing or glamour sustains personal and social well-being. In the first place, glamour is associated with the divine or religion, which is motivating for people's collective endeavor (Stewart et al. 2012). Glamour is also facilitative of leadership, conducive to people's compliance and deference (Goss 2005; Torfing 1999; Zeidner et al. 2009). Notably, glamour is inspirational and morale building (Ardichvili 2001). Hence, glamour helps maintain cooperation (Mulroy 1997). Glamour is also a quality conducive to entrepreneurship (Alsord et al. 2004). In this vein, glamour helps institutionalization, which means setting institutions up for agreement, order, stability, economic activity, efficiency, networking, empowerment, norms, law, legislation, legitimacy, bureaucracy, sanctioning, enforcement, meaning, culture, organization, and practice (Lowndes and Roberts 2013; Nee 2005; Peters 1999; Scott 2008; Thornton et al. 2012). By facilitating institutionalization, glamour is hence a key to social integration and functioning. Essentially, glamour is power (Hallett 2007). Therefore, glamour is a guarantee of personal and social success.

Modeling means setting the idol as a model for learning, emulation, and/or identification. It upholds the primary function of fulfillment and the secondary function of latency. In meeting the function of fulfillment, modeling enables the realization of talents, as in learning from the model (Girsh 2014; Stevens 2010). Meanwhile, modeling also holds the function of latency by perpetuating values, norms, and other ideas (Raviv et al. 1996; C. Wang et al. 2009). As such, many idols become role models for people to satisfy their needs (Fraser and Brown 2002). The model idols tend to be appealing, talented, heroic, and moral (Kinsella et al. 2015a; Stever 2008). Desire for modeling is a crucial determinant of idolatry (Hoegele et al. 2014). Hence, modeling is rather inalienable from idolatry. Essentially, modeling is particularly prominent in Chinese culture, with reference to its Confucian tradition to learn to be virtuous from sages (Reed 1995).

In satisfying the functions of fulfillment and latency, modeling appears to be salutary to the person and beneficial to society. Notably, modeling fosters body esteem or a positive body image through learning relevant norms and practices and thus, helps in grooming oneself like the idols (Katz-Wise et al. 2013). For practice in general, modeling contributes to self-efficacy (Bradley et al. 2000). Self-efficacy is certainly a component of well-being and thus sustains self-esteem, optimism, satisfaction, and quality of life, and conversely dampens anger, anxiety, depression, and negative affect (Luszczynska and Gutierrez-Dona 2005). Furthermore, self-efficacy is conducive to achievement, which can be socially beneficial (Luszczynska and Gutierrez-Dona 2005). Similarly, modeling teaches sustained mastery, power, or empowerment (Kezar and Moriatry 2000). Mastery is another component of well-being and reduces pressure and depression (Conger and Conger 2002). Furthermore, modeling attachment, socializing, caring, social acceptance, or favorable social interaction directly contributes to well-being (Lopez et al. 2014). For instance, modeling oneself on parents could facilitate sociability (Engels et al. 2001). Sociability, in turn, sustains self-esteem and belonging and alleviates distress or strain (Anderson-Butcher et al. 2008; De Bruyn and Boom 2005; Larson et al. 2007). Sociability certainly helps in making friends, which is also a benefit from modeling (Parade et al. 2010). In the same way, modeling is conducive to marriage in that it is a way of learning about how to be married (Starrels and Holm 2000). Particularly, modeling on idols is a way to learn about romantic love (Wan 1997). Modeling also invites social support from others (Bernardon et al. 2011). Moreover, sociability contributes to work competence, which is socially beneficial (Collins and van Dulmen 2006). Self-esteem also directly benefits from modeling, such as that on peers, to maintain self-esteem by showing lovability (Hendry et al. 1993; Song et al. 2009; Turner and Scherman 1996). Obviously, such modeling reduces social anxiety and isolation and provides security to further attachment and flourishing (Cotterell 2007). For instance, security fosters self-efficacy and coping and diminished depression (Lopez and Gormley 2002). This echoes the contribution of modeling found in the area of health (Abada et al. 2007). Having resourceful people to model themselves on thus counts as an asset for youth development (Kegler et al. 2005; King and Benson 2005). Particularly, modeling on family can be a developmental benefit (Thomas 2001). Modeling thus represents a way of learning for development (Tan 1986). An important aspect of development is that for citizenship, which benefits from modeling (Kahne et al. 2006).

Moreover, modeling such as that on family encourages cognitive development by stimulating thinking (Bradley et al. 2000). Correspondingly, modeling is instrumental to moral development, which is associated with cognitive development (Hoffman 2000; Lapsley 1996). In a similar vein, modeling such as that on adults also helps prosocial development (Scales et al. 2000). Another cognitive or intellectual benefit of modeling is increased creativity (Simonton 1978).

Modeling is also facilitative of career development in consolidating career motives, goals, and aspirations (Flouri and Buchanan 2002). Similarly, modeling on parents raises educational aspirations (Hao and Bonstead-Bruns 1998). Such development usually benefits from modeling on parents (Stringer and Kerpelman 2010). Modeling is also responsible for academic or educational success, including learning and its strategies (Schunk and Zimmerman 1996). Meanwhile, the success of civic education, moral education, or character education hinges on modeling (Arthur 2008; Berkowitz et al. 2008; Joseph and Efron 2005; Kahne and Middaugh 2009). Modeling in such education can motivate people to strive for the good and for true understanding and can relieve distress (Kristjansson 2006). Essentially, educational modeling stems from the Confucian tradition prevailing in Chinese culture (Wang 2004; S. Zhang 2003). This tradition advocates modeling for comprehensive, whole-person education and development (Huang 1998). In the West, modeling represents a kind of cognitive apprenticeship in education (Furnham-Diggory 1992). In addition, modeling on parents or teachers can prevent externalizing problems, prostitution, and gang involvement (Bradley et al. 2000; Cusick 2002; Lussier et al. 2002; Taylor et al. 2003). Modeling thereby represents an important preventive means against youth problems (Brennan and Shaw 2015). Modeling is also an effective means for programs for youth development, empowerment, or problem prevention (McWhirter 1994; Tan 1986). In this scenario, service organizers would serve as models (Youniss and Yates 1997). Hence, modeling on prosocial or conventional figures is beneficial to youth and society in terms of education, moral development, career development, problem prevention, and flourishing.

Commodifying of the idol means subscription to the idol's materials, typically commodities for possession, consumption, maintaining contact, and/or adoring (Schultze et al. 1991; Wang et al. 2009). It fulfills the adaptation function of getting material or tangible benefits from idols' videos, shows, photos, books, clothing, paraphernalia, and others. In this regard, it is compatible with the commercial economy or market and its consumerism (Fairchild 2007; Girsh 2014; Schee et al. 2013; Stevens 2010). It thereby satisfies the hedonic need to derive pleasure from consumption (Buxton 1983). Accordingly, commodifying or consumption of idol-related materials is satisfying by catering to the empty self, characterized by depression, isolation, self-disrespect, and obsession for individualism (Reeves et al. 2012). Commodifying of the idol also serves to reduce the distance from the idol (Radford and Bloch 2012). It particularly characterizes fandom as a form of idolatry (Radford and Bloch 2012).

Essentially, commodification simply fits consumer society nowadays (Bauman 2005). Commodification or the market is valuable because of the decline in social support in modern society (Holt 1997). Moreover, youth need to use commodification or subscription to certain idols to express optimal distinctiveness (Berger and Heath 2008). That is, commodification is germane to identity making or maintenance (Croghan et al. 2006; Kawamura 2006; Valentine 1999; Zukin 1998). Such a fabricated identity, nonetheless, is conducive to social inclusion (Croghan et al. 2006). At the same time, commodification is affordable because of socioeconomic development in society and youth (Gershuny 2000). Such development also consolidates bureaucratization, rationalization, efficiency, calculability, predictability, and control about commodification and thus facilitates commodification (Ritzer et al. 2001). Notably, development of the culture industry encourages the commodification of idols (Ritzer et al. 2001). Commodification thereby appeals to the modern or postmodern lifestyle that compares, uses, and savors commodities (Glennie 1998; O'Boyle 2005). Hence, commodification helps form a subculture regarding the commodity or idol that has its own norms, traditions, and adherents (Kawamura 2006). Furthermore, commodification seems inevitable, with the rise of innovation, information, the market, and consumer sovereignty (Firat and Dholakia 1998). Under such conditions, commodification or consumption is more important than production, as is prominent in postmodern society (Crompton 1996; Kawamura 2006). Consequently, commodification has drawn much policy concern about pricing, promotion, and communication regarding commodification (Campbell 2004). Commodification is also integral to neoliberalist policy that advocates economic or market activities (Trentmann 2007).

In satisfying the adaptation function of gaining materially, commodifying or consumption is evidently satisfactory. In the first place, commodifying or consumption means the intake of resources or energy and thus is energizing for various strivings that are helpful to the person and society (Ekstrom and Ostman 2013; Kahne et al. 2013a). Commodifying can also make one knowledgeable, at least about the commodity (Ekstrom and Ostman 2013). This is not surprising as commodifying can instigate studying (Marazyan 2011). With the enhancement of knowledge, commodifying can build trust, interest, and involvement (Ekstrom and Ostman 2013; Hooghe et al. 2015). Furthermore, commodifying can establish social status (Roberts 1998). Eventually, commodifying can make one proactive and competitive through energizing and empowering (Lever et al. 2005). Overall, commodifying can be a means to sustain well-being (Wang and VanderWeele 2011). It raises positive affect such as pride and reduced negative affect such as shame (Hudders and Pandelaere 2012). This reflects the arousal effect of commodifying (Wang et al. 2010). Commodifying of culture, as in fandom, is also conducive to life satisfaction (Bourdieu 1979; Roberts et al. 2001).

Faming of the idol means regarding the idol as famous. In other words, faming means honoring or acclaiming the idol. It fulfills the primary function of adaptation and the secondary function of integration for socializing or basking in reflected glory, respectively. Faming reflects the desire for or interest in prestige (Greenberg et al. 2010; Holub et al. 2008; Noser and Zeighler-Hill 2014; Southard and Zeigler-Hill 2016). Fame can cover the lifestyle, altruism, and drive (Southard and Zeigler-Hill 2016). Typically, faming applies to stars (De Backer 2012). Fame is also a determinant of idolatry because of the ease of recognition of the idol (De Becker 2012). As such, desire for fame upholds idolatry (Gountas et al. 2012).

In realizing its functions, faming can be salutary to the person and beneficial to society. In the first place, the faming individual can earn fame by basking in reflected glory (Preckel and Brull 2010). Fame, as earned, can be salutary, salubrious, or wholesome in sustaining health, probably because of conformity to social norms about healthy habits (Al-krenawi et al. 2011; Emerson and Hatton 2007; Lichtenstein et al. 1999; Thomas 1997). For instance, fame can be conducive to participation in sport, which sustains health (van de Werfhorst and Kraaykamp 2001). As such, fame can contribute to life satisfaction (Al-krenawi et al. 2011; Appleton and Song 2008). Moreover, fame can contribute to satisfaction with justice, including procedural justice, in society (Tyler et al. 1997; Whyte and Gao 2009). Fame can also help sustain self-efficacy and self-esteem (Al-krenawi et al. 2011; Caplan and Schooler 2007). Fame also contributes to society by activating civic or political interest, participation, and engagement (Pattie et al. 2004; van de Werfhorst and Kraaykamp 2001). Similarly, fame tends to contribute to work involvement (Mulder and Wagner 1998). As such, fame can sustain mastery or competence (Oldmeadow and Fiske 2007). Fame can also help family functioning (Al-krenawi et al. 2011). Furthermore, fame can sustain humor and thus social functioning (Martin 2007). In addition, fame can help individuals to restrain anger (Stets and Tsushima 2001). Hence, fame can facilitate social interaction (Liebler and Sandefur 2002). Furthermore, fame can lead to volunteering (Wilson 2000). Overall, fame guides healthy and moral practices to sustain personal and social functioning, which is contributory to society.

Romanticizing of the idol means attributing romance and lovability to the idol for loving or infatuation (Fetscherin and Santa Barbara 2014; Wan 1997). This form of idolizing caters to the primary function of integration and the secondary function of maintaining social well-being and realizing personal wishes, respectively. Accordingly, romanticizing sustains a social or parasocial relationship and satisfies the need for love and affirming personal attractiveness or lovability. As such, romanticizing is the extension of self-love to the idol (Lin and Lin 2007). Essentially, romanticizing seems to reflect a feminine practice (Adams-Price and Greene 1990; Argyle 1994; Greene and Adams-Price 1990). This means maintaining affiliation or intimacy with the romanticized idol. Romanticizing tends to be easy and common, as it emphasizes something erotic but superficial in the idol (Alexander 2010). As such, romanticizing appears to be a constituent of idolatry (Schindler et al. 2015). Furthermore, romanticizing seems to be a norm in idolatry, because it is safe in the sense of not involving an actual social relationship (Karniol 2001).

Romanticizing can contribute to personal and social functioning through creating an experience of love or intimacy. The experience is beneficial because it provides the object for maintaining a relationship and attachment (Arseth et al. 2009). It is salutary in establishing identity and belongingness (Mooney et al. 2007). Evidently, romanticizing or love contributes to well-being (Steger et al. 2006). A clear instance is the contribution of romanticizing to satisfaction with romantic relations (Tsou and Liu 2001). In a similar vein, romanticizing in the family champions family well-being (Chuang 2005). More broadly, romanticizing in any relation maintains the quality of the relation (Jackson et al. 2006). In addition, romanticizing as a way of forming lovability and attachment buttresses resilience (Shaver and Mikulincer 2012). Romanticizing also contributes to well-being through elevating positive affect, which is useful in broadening and building strategies to sustain well-being (Parks et al. 2014). Conversely, romanticizing reduces depression through upholding lovability (Busch 2009). For the benefit of society, romanticizing can contribute to cooperation, at least with the loved one (Sanderson 2001). Romanticizing can also prevent problem behavior, including doping (McCarthy and Casey 2008). Notably, romanticizing can prevent criminal or delinquent behavior because of the development of moral sensitivity rather than psychopathy or antisociality (Jones 2016). Romanticizing or finding love with others therefore benefits the person and society, such as through prevention of crime.

Befriending of the idol means regarding the idol as a friend, typically with warmth, sociability, and amity, to maintain contact, conversation, interaction, friendship, attachment, and even intimacy (Holub et al. 2008). It is the forging of a parasocial relationship, which is imagined and one-sided, with the idol (Cole and Leets 1998; Giles 2000; Giles and Maltby 2004; Gleason et al. 2017; McCutcheon et al. 2003). This is a platonic relationship or attachment (Adams-Price and Greene 1990). Befriending also treats the idol as a teacher or family member to fabricate intimacy (White and O'Brien 1999). Same-sex befriending is important here for visualizing support, validation, and modeling from the idol friend (Feldman and Wentzel 1995; Lempers and Clark-Lempers 1993). Befriending has the typical properties of maintaining closeness, proximity, communication, familiarity, security, and trust (Cole and Leets 1999; Cotterell 1992; Ellison 1991; Hafner 2009; Larose and Boivin 1998; Raja et al. 1992). Familiarizing oneself with the idol, and thus understanding the idol and imagining inclusion by the idol, are central to befriending (Hafner 2009). The befriended idol is likely to be a hero who is helpful (Sweetman et al. 2013).

Befriending is beneficial through attachment and the security it breeds (Burgess et al. 2006). The benefit typically happens in the growth of self-esteem and development in identity (Burgess et al. 2006; Wu and Wong 2013). Befriending can also uphold self-efficacy and reduce anxiety, depression, and psychological symptoms (Arseth et al. 2009; Brendgen et al. 2000; Henderson et al. 2009). Furthermore, befriending can contribute to belongingness, relational competence, and reduced loneliness (Brendgen et al. 2000; Henderson et al. 2009; Zysberg 2012). Befriending can also sustain self-control and moral and prosocial behavior (Benda 2002; Elliott et al. 2005; Walker and Frimer 2009; Wu and Wong 2013). Moreover, befriending is conducive to sociability (Barry and Wigfield 2002). Befriending is also instrumental to school attachment, academic achievement, and employment (Benson 2007; Franklin 1995; Moody and White 2003; Morgan and Sorensen 1999; Mortimer et al. 2003). In addition, befriending can prevent externalizing problems, dropping out of school, theft, and delinquent involvement (Elliott et al. 2005; Haynie 2001; McCarthy et al. 2004;

Staff and Kraeger 2008). Through creating a feeling of security, befriending can foster sharing and togetherness as opposed to argument (Monteoliva et al. 2016). Overall, befriending or intimacy is salutary (Ramsey and Gentzler 2015). It is also beneficial to society through prosocial, moral, and other conventional practices.

Popularizing the idol means regarding the idol as popular, notably among significant others. The idol is likely to be a star (Argyle 1994; X. He 2006; Sobel 1981). Popularizing represents conforming to the norm of idolatry, particularly among significant others (Lindenberg et al. 2011). Hence, popularizing implies maintaining relationships among significant others and the idol (Adams-Price and Greene 1990). This illustrates the solid integration function of popularizing for relationship building among people. An instance of the integration function happens in gossiping about the idol, which means sharing information and norms and thus upholding unity among people (De Becker et al. 2007). It may be salient more in girls than in boys (He and Feng 2002).

Popularizing or conformity appears to be functional to the person and society. Essentially, popularizing is important in socialization, involving training and learning (Cohen and Prinstein 2006). Popularizing can contribute to goal setting, including mastery and performance, and to receiving support or guidance from others to sustain well-being (Jiang et al. 2015). Thus, popularizing is facilitative of relationship building (Hendry et al. 1993). Popularizing is also conducive to tolerance, which is favorable to democratic social functioning (Feldman 2003; Finkel and Ernst 2005). At the same time, popularizing particularly fits collectivist culture, and is satisfactory and functional to the person and society, notably in maintaining a loyal or moral life (Bush et al. 2002; T. Chang et al. 2015; Soenens et al. 2012). Moreover, popularizing is a desirable property for youth development in order to sustain duties and social order (Ellenwood 2007). Popularizing or conformity therefore underlies fitness and functioning for the person and society.

Personalizing the idol means finding an idol to fit one's personal characteristics or preference. This style of idolizing indicates the importance of personal interest in idolatry (Maltby et al. 2004b). It illustrates that idolatry is individualistic, individuating, and distinctive to establish identity (Lin and Lin 2007; Madhavan and Crowell 2014; Maltby et al. 2006; Stevens 2010). At least, it reflects an exploration for identity (Adams-Price and Greene 1990). In other words, personalizing registers self-expansion in consolidating and exhibiting the self (Schindler et al. 2015). In all, personalizing identifies the latency function of personality maintenance and development. Personalizing is thus a basis for idolatry (Reeves et al. 2012).

Personalizing can be salutary to the persona and beneficial to society. Principally, personalizing represents self-understanding or self-consciousness (Hoffman 2014). Moreover, personalizing is required for adaptation and development for independent living (Tricarico 2016). Development entails empathy, deference, and ability to predict (Branner and Nilsen 2005; Kruse and Walper 2008). Such development can be the basis for competence, self-efficacy,

Table 6.3 Factor loadings on four idolizing factors

Item	Glorifying	Prizing	Modeling	Popularizing
Glamourizing	.707	.305	.128	−.015
Beautifying	.594	.267	−.107	.089
Faming	.588	.179	.251	.140
Crediting	.481	.118	.235	.051
Commodifying	.209	.701	.091	.020
Idealizing	.206	.569	.372	.030
Befriending	.283	.487	.395	−.064
Romanticizing	.325	.464	.075	.137
Personalizing	.223	.249	.175	−.237
Modeling	.122	.205	.867	−.002
Popularizing	.192	.091	.030	.803

self-esteem, and work orientation (Kruse and Walper 2008). Personalizing can create motivation, which in turn can sustain achievement, such as academic achievement (Lew et al. 1998). As such, personalizing is conducive to learning (Short et al. 1992). Generally, personalizing can thereby buttress competence, effort, and performance (Patall et al. 2008), which are beneficial to the person and society through personal work.

Glorifying of the idol is a composite of glamourizing, beautifying, faming, and crediting of the idol, resulting from factor analysis in this study (elaborated later) (Table 6.3). Hence, glorifying assigns glory to the idol to shine with glamour, beauty, handsomeness, or attractiveness, fame, and success. In other words, the glorified idol is able, skillful, striving, appealing, attractive, sexy, energetic, glamorous, successful, prestigious, and/or renowned (De Backer 2012; Gleason et al. 2017; Greenberg et al. 2010; Madhavan and Crowell 2014; Noser and Zeigler-Hill 2014; Robinson et al. 2016; Rusch et al. 2015; Sarapin et al. 2015; Schindler et al. 2013; Southard and Zeigler-Hill 2016). Generally, glorifying caters to the fulfillment function of realizing people's talents or treasurable qualities.

Prizing of the idol is another idolizing factor emerging from the study to subsume commodifying, idealizing, befriending, and romanticizing. Thus, prizing means finding values in the idol to extol. The prized idol or its material would be moral, principled, helpful, altruistic, selfless, protective, close, intimate, honest, trustworthy, affectionate, authentic, consumable, and saleable (Fraser and Brown 2002; Kinsella et al. 2015b; Madhavan and Crowell 2014; Maltby et al. 2008; Radford and Bloch 2012; Sarapin et al. 2015; Schlenker et al. 2008; Sweetman et al. 2013). Generally, prizing meets the adaptation function of acquiring valuable resources from the idol.

Idol roles or identities

The idol can take any of the following characteristics or identities: Western, Japanese, Chinese, female, male, entertaining, athletic, academic, ideological, literary, political, military, business, historical, fictional, nonfictional, familial, heroic, altruistic, idealistic, musical, mathematical, professional, artistic, navigating, or parent, teacher, peer, criminal, star, luminary, celebrity, and/or noncelebrity. These roles or identities realize the functions of fulfillment, adaptation, integration, and latency with respect to the functionalist perspective.

Among the roles or identities, the hero is prominent. Within heroes, the celebrity, athlete, and politician are representative in descending order (Madhavan and Crowell 2014). The hero is likely to be a leader who is energizing and advising (Allison and Goethals 2016). The worshipper is energized by basking in reflected glory to elevate his or her morality, reverence, and admiration and to maintain physical and mental health, including self-esteem. All these benefits entail or reflect energy input. In advising, the hero establishes a deep role and deep time, which are substantive experiences to raise and consolidate the worshipper's intelligence and wisdom that transcends ordinary rationality. Accordingly, the hero vividly and intensely illustrates what is good or ethical to ponder and do. For instance, the hero can show what and for what to sacrifice, even though the sacrifice is irrational. The hero also reveals vicissitudes in life for learning and endurance. Moreover, the hero has such qualities as action orientation, authenticity, instrumentality, intelligence, perseverance, likability, nurturance, beneficence, power, self-creation, having principles, offering protection, and, typically, being male (Balswick and Ingoldsby 1992; Calvert et al. 2004; Fraser and Brown 2002; Greenwood 2007; Holub et al. 2008; Schlenker et al. 2008).

Obviously, the hero is heroic in being altruistic, selfless, helpful, prosocial, convicted, courageous, determined, honest, inspiring, modeling, moral, saving, risk taking, and sociable (Franco et al. 2011; Kinsella et al. 2015a, 2015b). The sociable characteristics include adventuring, exploring, and leading as well as being political and ethical, such as through whistleblowing (Franco et al. 2011). Furthermore, the hero displays caring, fathering, charisma, reliability, resilience, smartness, leadership, romance, self-control, and physical strength, such as being muscled and exercising (Goethals and Allison 2012). The hero is also likely to be trendy and transcendent across time and space (Goethals and Allison 2012). As such, the hero is desirable for affiliation or attachment (North et al. 2005). Nevertheless, the hero can be an underdog, martyr, bureaucrat, and even a dying person, who can also attract sympathy, pity, and eventually respect and emulation (Franco et al. 2011; Goethals and Allison 2012). The hero is vital because of the need and function of heroizing or hero making (Franco et al. 2011). Accordingly, people need elevation and recognition, which the hero can instantiate and exemplify. Usually, the hero has some similarities with the worshipper and thus represents the ideal projected by the worshipper (Schlenker et al. 2008).

The hero has shown his or her functions for the benefit of the worshipper and society. These functions include motivating the worshipper to take initiative, behave morally, care about social problems, find meaning in life, and avoid delinquent involvement (Cao and Wang 1993; Ibarra and Kitsuse 2003; Larson 2000;

Solomon 2003; Youniss and Yates 1999). That is, the hero shows the worshipper how to exercise self-control and contribute to others or society.

Celebrities, as famous people, are prominent among idols and heroes (Fraser and Brown 2002; Houran et al. 2005; Madhavan and Crowell 2014; Maltby et al. 2004; Price et al. 2014; Reeves et al. 2012; Sivami et al. 2010). The celebrity tends to be snobbish, pretentious, prominent in the media, image building, and attention drawing (Fraser and Brown 2002; North et al. 2005). Moreover, the celebrity is likely to be attractive, beautiful, princess-like, lovable, sublime, and/or cool (Alexander 2010). Worship of the celebrity is prone to be irrational (Alexander 2010). Crucially, the celebrity represents the paragon for idolatry, such that idolatry highly depends on the availability of the celebrity (Livingstone et al. 2007). As such, involvement with the celebrity is a sufficient determinant of idolatry (Yurchisin et al. 2009). In other words, celebrities arise to manipulate people and thus lead to their celebrity worship and fetishism, especially with the advent of postmodernity (Alexander 2010). In China, many celebrities function to advocate and inculcate nationalism (Liu and Berkowitz 2014).

The celebrity is functional to and influential on the person and society (Hsiao 2004). Accordingly, the celebrity can contribute to the civic efficacy of the youth worshipper (Wen and Cui 2014). In addition, the celebrity can reduce the political apathy of the youth worshipper (Austin et al. 2008). The celebrity can draw worshippers' attention to much information, as disclosed through the Internet (Livingstone et al. 2007).

More specifically, celebrities include athletes, performers, and newscasters (De Becker 2012; White and Molina 2016). The most eminent ones are stars (Argyle 1994; De Becker 2012). They share the common feature of reliance on the media, which excel in grooming and propagating information about idols (Fraser and Brown 2002; Lin and Lin 2007). Nevertheless, their eminence tends to be transient (Smith and Wright 2000). Star worship or star idolatry is likely to be the most prominent or well-known form of idolatry (De Becker 2012).

Models or role models are cognate or have much overlap with idols (Fraser and Brown 2002). Typically, models are teachers, parents, other relatives, friends, acquaintances, and celebrities in descending order of possibility (Sjaastad 2012). They are functional in fulfilling their followers' need and tend to be enduringly important to their followers (Fraser and Brown 2002). Modeling on or regarding a decent person as a model can be functional in sustaining self-efficacy, mastery, empathy or consideration, prosociality, creativity, and leadership (Kezar and Moriarty 2000; Scales et al. 2000; Simonton 1978; Stringer and Kerpelman 2010). Furthermore, modeling can be conducive to furthering education aspirations, self-regulated learning, academic achievement, and career motivation (Flouri and Buchanan 2002; Hao and Bonstead-Bruns 1998; Schunk and Zimmerman 1996; Simonton 1994). In addition, such modeling can impede externalizing behavior and delinquent involvement, including prostitution and violence (Bradley et al. 2000; Cusick 2002; Hurd et al. 2011; Taylor et al. 2003).

Correlating idolizing with self-efficacy, attachment, intimacy, and idol characteristics

Showing correlates with idolizing is a way to elucidate idolizing. Potential correlates for examination include self-efficacy, attachment styles, and intimacy factors, as well as acceptance of the idol and model and the idol's roles or identities. Attachment styles comprise secure attachment, preoccupied attachment, dismissive attachment, and fearful attachment. Intimacy factors encompass frank intimacy, sensitive intimacy, attaching intimacy, exclusive intimacy, sharing intimacy, imposing intimacy, partnering intimacy, and trusting intimacy. Furthermore, the correlates can differ between boys and girls, between early adolescents and older adolescents, and between the Mainland Chinese youth and Hong Kong Chinese youth.

Self-efficacy refers to belief in one's own ability to achieve or to tackle problems generally (Bhanot and Jovanovic 2009). It registers one's power and social-cognitive functioning, including self-organizing, self-reflection, self-regulation, and judging (Hirschi 2009; Luszczynska and Gutierrez-Dona 2005). The efficacy, power, or functioning is primarily conducive to action in terms of, representing, or leading to exploration, investment, participation, engagement, prevention, management, self-regulation, and achievement in various fields (Baartman and Ruijs 2011; Fahmy 2006; Levpuscek et al. 2009; Luszczynska and Gutierrez-Dona 2005; McMahon et al. 2015; Rogers and Creed 2011; Schnell et al. 2015; Walker et al. 2006). Conversely, self-efficacy forestalls indecision and problem behavior such as smoking (Carvajal et al. 2004; Fosco and Feinberg 2015; Guay et al. 2006). Self-efficacy can also contribute to optimism, resiliency, entrepreneurship, and general skill acquisition (Fortune et al. 2005; Luszczynska and Guticrrez-Dona 2005; Milioni et al. 2015; Pinquart et al. 2004; Rawlings 2012; Schmitt-Redermund and Vondracek 2002). Furthermore, self-efficacy underlies motivation, orientation, expectation, aspiration, and intention of many behaviors (Armitage et al. 1999; DiRenzo et al. 2013; Eccles et al. 2000; Johnston and White 2003; Luszczynska and Gutierrez-Dona 2005; Turner et al. 2004). Self-efficacy can also foster favorable attitudes toward career, school, sport, and many others (Creed and Patton 2003; Faircloth and Hamm 2005; Rogers and Creed 2011; Turner et al. 2004; T. Wu et al. 2003). Eventually, self-efficacy can buttress feelings of well-being such as satisfaction, self-esteem, and evaluation of life quality, school, career, and others (Burger and Samuel 2017; Cikrikci and Odaci 2016; Luszczynska and Gutierrez-Dona 2005; Pinquart et al. 2004; Yon et al. 2012). In addition, self-efficacy can prevent anger, anxiety, depression, distress, and negative affect (Gore and Aseltine 1995; Fosco and Feinberg 2015; Luszczynska and Gutierrez-Dona 2005; Pinquart et al. 2004; Sheridan et al. 2015).

Attachment styles reflect beliefs in the internal mental working models crucial for social interaction and relationship building (Cotterell 2007). Obviously, attachment styles are primal, according to attachment theory, which prioritizes the influences of early life attachment experience and its product of attachment styles (Monteoliva et al. 2016). Accordingly, attachment means seeking and maintaining a close and proximate relationship (Cotterell 2007). Attachment developed in early life is particularly vital in shaping attachment styles evolving later. Apart from the usual component of attachment security during early life and later, attachment can take the form of insecure attachment, which comprises preoccupied attachment, dismissive attachment, and fearful attachment (Allen et al. 2005). Secure attachment means that the object or others are accessible or approachable and help to build a sense of security, confidence, and trust in the object or others. Dismissive attachment means that the object or others are rejecting and thus engendering insecurity. Fearful attachment means diffidence in securing a desired relationship. Preoccupied attachment means a high desire to pursue a rejected relationship. Secure attachment is important for championing independence, togetherness, and sharing, as opposed to argument and monotony (Monteoliva et al. 2016). Essentially, (secure) attachment buttresses social or friendship quality through encouragement of exploration (Markiewicz et al. 2001). By the same token, attachment upholds romantic quality (Giordano et al. 2001).

The contribution of attachment is empirically evident. Attachment is the basis for success, self-control, identity achievement, and well-being, including life satisfaction, adjustment, and self-esteem (Collins and Feeney 2000; Harter 2012; Kennedy 1999; Jiang et al. 2013; Lapsley and Edgerton 2002; Liu et al. 2010; Lopez et al. 2014; Meier and Allen 2008; Benda 2002; Richardson et al. 2015; Shen 2009; Song et al. 2009; Wyman 2003). Furthermore, attachment is conducive to friendship, intimacy, morality, prosociality, social competence, career exploration, and social support received (Benda 2002; Eberly and Montemayor 1998; Carlo et al. 2012; Engels et al. 2001; Markiewicz et al. 2001; Miller and Hoicoisitz 2004; Mohr et al. 2010; Parade et al. 2010; Vignoli et al. 2005; Walker and Frimer 2009). Importantly, attachment can prevent isolation, psychopathology, distress, anxiety, depression, doping, alcoholism, externalizing behavior, career anxiety, and career indecision (Benda 2002; Braunstein-Bercovitz et al. 2012; Choo and Shek 2013; Elliott et al. 2005; Gullone et al. 2006; Lussier et al. 2002; McCarthy and Casey 2008; Nishikawa et al. 2010; Shamir-Essakow et al. 2005; Tokar et al. 2003; Ward et al. 2006). Attachment to parents particularly sustains assertiveness, enjoyment, morality, empathy, leadership, self-efficacy, frustration tolerance, social relation, social integration, and task orientation (Buist et al. 2004; Carlo et al. 2012; Englund et al. 2000; Hay 2001; Marcos and Bahr 1988; Ridenour et al. 2006). At the same time, attachment to parents can reduce depression, anxiety, loneliness, delinquency, suicide, theft, violence, externalizing behavior, and association with delinquent peers (Augustyn and McGloin 2013; Bernardon et al. 2011; Costello and Vowell 1999; Fergusson et al. 2003; Graham and Easterbrooks 2000; Reynolds and Crea 2015; Ridenour et al. 2006; Shamir-Essakow et al. 2005; Strohschein and Matthew 2015; Warr 2005). Conversely, insecure, fearful attachment can impede motivation, individuation, intimacy, prosociality, social orientation, alliance building, romantic relationships, career motivation, and the reception of social support (Collins and Feeney 2000; Downing and Nauta 2010; Eggermant 2004; Erez et al. 2008; Leybman et al. 2011; Miller and Hoicoisitz 2004). Insecure attachment also foments loneliness, conflicts, identity diffusion, career anxiety, career indecision, and various other problems (Braunstein-Bercovitz et al. 2012; Downing and Nauta 2010; Gillath et al. 2005; Lapsley and Edgerton 2002; Tokar et al. 2003). Therefore, for youth, secure attachment is functional, and insecure attachment such as fearful attachment is dysfunctional.

Intimacy, as applied to the closest friend, means maintaining a close relationship. It tends to be a transient state in youth (Christopher et al. 2016). Intimate persons can be relatives, friends or best friends, romantic partners, and role models (Christopher et al. 2016; Henderson et al. 2009; Miller and Hoicoisitz 2004; S. Johnson et al. 2016; Zeng and Xie 2008). Intimacy is higher with parents than friends, other relatives, and other people in descending order (S. Johnson et al. 2016). In more detail, intimacy is composed of eight dimensions, namely, frank intimacy, sensitive intimacy, attaching intimacy, exclusive intimacy, sharing intimacy, imposing intimacy, partnering intimacy, and trustful intimacy. Frank intimacy means showing frankness, honesty, or self-disclosure. Sensitive intimacy involves care and responsiveness. Attaching intimacy means following and engaging. Exclusive intimacy entails rejecting other relationships. Sharing intimacy engages communication and mutuality. Imposing intimacy shows ordering and regulation. Partnering intimacy highlights companionship and togetherness. Trustful intimacy reveals faith and loyalty. Intimacy, including its various dimensions, is important or functional in view of attachment and object relations theories (Arseth et al. 2009). These theories posit that attachment and maintaining relations with objects or people are necessary to relieve uncertainty and stress and to fulfill the need for care (Jiang et al. 2013; Lopez et al. 2014).

Self-efficacy attachment (secure as opposed to insecure), and intimacy are crucial for scrutinizing the issue of spillover versus compensation in idolizing. According to the thesis of spillover, assimilation, or compatibility, idolizing maintains a positive correlation with self-efficacy belief, secure attachment, and intimacy with friends or other significant people (Huang and Mitchell 2014). This thesis states that favor for one spills over to favor for another. By contrast, the thesis of compensation, contrast, contradiction, or conflict posits that idolizing holds a negative correlation with self-efficacy belief, secure attachment, and intimacy (Argyle 1994; Engle and Kasser 2005; Feldman and Wentzel 1995; Jenson 1992; Seiffge-Krenke 1997). This thesis asserts that idolizing is a compensation for inadequate social relationships. Both spillover and compensation theses are plausible in light of existing theory and evidence as follows.

Correlations between idolizing and self-efficacy

A positive correlation between idolizing and self-efficacy manifests assimilation, expansion, generalizing, or spillover between idolizing and self-efficacy. That is, when idolizing is high, self-efficacy is also high and vice versa. By contrast, a negative correlation between idolizing and self-efficacy implies contrast, compensating, conflict, or contradiction between idolizing and self-efficacy. That is, when idolizing is high, self-efficacy is low and vice versa.

Positive correlation

Idolizing of a figure is likely to secure a positive correlation with self-efficacy under five conditions: First, the self and idol have an overlap. Second, self-efficacy causes idolizing. Third, idolizing causes self-efficacy. Fourth, idolizing and self-efficacy share a common cause. Fifth, idolizing and self-efficacy have a common consequence.

Idolizing of a figure is likely to hold a positive correlation with self-efficacy simply because the figure is similar or tantamount to the self. One possibility is that the idolized figure is a self-created product based on the projection of oneself (Fraser and Brown 2002). In addition, the figure is likely to be similar to the idolizer in many respects (Schlenker et al. 2008). Similarity is likely to originate from the idolizer's wishful thinking (Konijn et al. 2007). Thus, the idolizer identifies very much with the idol and even treats the idol as an extension of himself or herself (Huang and Mitchell 2014). As such, idolizing is the expansion of the idolizer's self to incorporate the idol (Schindler et al. 2015). This underlies overlapping between the idol and self (Huang and Mitchell 2014).

Self-efficacy is likely to cause idolizing, thus culminating in a positive correlation with idolizing. This is possible when self-esteem, which generally represents self-efficacy, shows a positive effect on idolizing (Seiffge-Krenke 1997; J. Turner 1993). A possible explanation is that self-efficacy may lead to the development of personal and social identity regarding efficacy, and this identity prompts identification with and thereby adoration of an idol, who is likely to be efficacious and thus have the same social identity (Adams 1985; Furnham 1990; C. Wang et al. 2009). In other words, idolatry results from self-expansion, which means expanding the self to cover an idol with equally high self-efficacy (Huang and Mitchell 2014).

Idolizing is also likely to cause self-efficacy, hence sustaining a positive correlation with self-efficacy. It is possible through the building of real, online, or parasocial social networking, which is conducive to self-efficacy (Fletcher et al. 2006; Moriarty 1992). Learning from or modeling on the idol, who is likely efficacious, is a possible mechanism for the contribution of idolizing to self-efficacy (Adams 1985; Moseley and Utley 2008).

Idolizing and self-efficacy are also likely to have a positive correlation due to their susceptibility to common causes. One condition is autonomy or self-determination, which is likely to underlie both idolizing and self-efficacy (Giles and Maltby 2004; S. To et al. 2014). Moreover, political interest and involvement appear to be common causes of both idolizing and self-efficacy (Austin et al. 2008).

Idolizing and self-efficacy can hold a positive correlation due to their common impacts on such consequences as belongingness, loyalty, fidelity, and/or compliance (Bush et al. 2005; Durlak et al. 2007; Faircloth and Hamm 2005;

Fetscherin and Barbara 2014). Meanwhile, both idolizing and self-efficacy have been shown to contribute to violence and criminality (Erdley and Asher 1996; Sheridan et al. 2007).

Negative correlation

Idolizing of a figure is likely to display a negative correlation with self-efficacy under five conditions: First, the self and idol are different and even adversarial. Second, self-efficacy impedes idolizing. Third, idolizing impairs self-efficacy. Fourth, idolizing and self-efficacy are susceptible to contradictory causes. Fifth, idolizing and self-efficacy engender contradictory consequences.

Idolizing of a figure and self-efficacy can maintain a negative correlation because the idol and self can be adversarial to each other. Accordingly, the idol would be the ideal model, adviser, or teacher to confront, instruct, and modify the self (Adams-Price and Greene 1990; Greenwood 2007; Reeves et al. 2012; Sjaastad 2012). That is, the idol can reveal the inadequacy of the self (Reeves et al. 2012). The idol is thus a contrast to the self for the self to reflect and improve. This happens especially when the idol is perfect, holy, sacred, saint-like, or adorable (He 2006). In addition, the idol tends to be a selfless person (Kinsella et al. 2015b). All these would distance the self from the idol.

Idolizing can diminish because of self-efficacy, thus sustaining a negative correlation between them. Principally, idolizing can work as a compensation for self-inefficacy (Jenson 1992). Moreover, idolizing supposedly happens because of the emptiness of self, as indicated by self-inefficacy (Reeves et al. 2012). Idolizing may therefore function to restore or enhance self-efficacy (Allison and Goethals 2010; Hoegele et al. 2014). Moreover, idolizing an idol, who is likely efficacious, may be a threat to self-efficacy because of social comparison (Adams 1985; Fosco and Feinberg 2015).

Idolizing can dampen self-efficacy, thus bolstering a negative correlation between them. In this connection, idolizing appears to impede creativity, critical thinking, adjustment, and satisfaction (Houran et al. 2005; Scharf and Levy 2015). These abilities and emotions, meanwhile, prop up self-efficacy (Hirschi 2009; Salavera et al. 2017). An explanation is that idolizing results from an empty self, which involves self-inefficacy (Reeves et al. 2012).

Idolizing and self-efficacy can exhibit a negative correlation because of contradictory causes that hold negative correlations. That is, the causes would have opposite effects on idolizing and self-efficacy. Accordingly, satisfaction can reduce idolizing but champion self-efficacy (Mortimer 2003; Reeves et al. 2012). Moreover, whereas stress and threat can reduce self-efficacy, they can raise idolizing (Dupree et al. 2007; Moriarty 1992). What is more, whereas social skill and attachment security are conducive to self-efficacy, they attenuate idolizing (Giles and Maltby 2004; Salavera et al. 2017). Similarly, whereas resiliency and flexibility sustain self-efficacy, they dampen idolizing (Maltby et al. 2004; Milioni et al. 2015). In addition, whereas socioeconomic status bolsters self-efficacy, it reduces idolizing (Argyle 1994; Mortimer 2003).

Accordingly, idolizing tends to be a compensation for socioeconomic failure (Argyle 1994).

Idolizing and self-efficacy can manifest a negative correlation when they exert opposite impacts on some consequences. Concerning well-being, whereas self-efficacy sustains satisfaction and adjustment, idolizing impairs them (Burger and Samuel 2017; Cikrikci and Odaci 2016; Pinquart et al. 2004; Scharf and Levy 2015). Conversely, whereas self-efficacy impedes anger, anxiety, depression, distress, guilt, and negative affect generally, idolizing maintains them (Fosco and Feinberg 2015; Gore and Aseltine 1995; Luszczynska and Gutierrez-Dona 2005; Moriarty 1992; Pinquart et al. 2004; Sheridan et al. 2015). Concerning behavioral consequences, whereas self-efficacy reduces problem behavior and criminality, idolizing foments them (Carvajal et al. 2004; Fosco and Feinberg 2015; Sheridan et al. 2007).

Correlations between idolizing and secure attachment

A positive correlation between idolizing and secure attachment style registers assimilation, expansion, generalizing, or spillover between idolizing and secure attachment style. That is, when idolizing is high, attachment style is also high and vice versa. This also means that idolizing has a negative correlation with insecure attachment style, fearful attachment, dismissive attachment, and preoccupied attachment. By contrast, a negative correlation between idolizing and secure attachment style signals contrast, compensating, conflict, or contradiction between idolizing and secure attachment style. That is, when idolizing is high, intimacy is low and vice versa. This also means that idolizing has a positive correlation with insecure attachment style, fearful attachment, dismissive attachment, and preoccupied attachment.

Positive correlation

Idolizing of a figure is likely to sustain positive correlations with secure attachment styles or negative correlations with insecure attachment styles, including secure attachment, preoccupied attachment, dismissive attachment, and fearful attachment. Such correlations are explicable in five ways: First, the figure idolized is simply a special case of a person targeted for attachment. At least, there is much overlap between the idol and the target for attachment. Moreover, idolizing and attachment are similar concepts, showing a positive relationship with the target of idolizing or attachment. Second, secure attachment style causes idolizing. Third, idolizing reinforces secure attachment style. Fourth, idolizing and secure attachment style are under the influences of some common causes. Fifth, idolizing and secure attachment have common consequences.

Idolizing of a figure displays positive correlations with secure attachment style, likely because of overlap between the idolized figure and people targeted for attachment in general. Clearly, idols can be people with talents; achievement; heroism; merit; morality; fame; charm; popularity; stardom; media exposure;

modeling quality; cultural capital, including orientations, knowledge, and skills fitting to a culture; or familial relationship with the idolizer (Calvert et al. 2001; Fraser and Brown 2002; Girsh 2014; S. Ryu et al. 2007; Schlenker et al. 2008; Shen 2001). Hence, the idol is very likely to be a target for personal attachment. Moreover, attachment is clearly a manifestation of idolizing, in terms of romanticizing or befriending (Cole and Leets 1999; Greene and Adams-Price 1990). Accordingly, the idol for attachment is trustworthy, desirable for communication, and capable of providing security (Cotterell 1992; de Jong 1992; Larose and Boivin 1998; Raja et al. 1992).

Another likely reason that idolizing and secure attachment style maintain positive correlations is because of the positive influences of the attachment style on idolizing. In theory, secure attachment style is a determinant of idolizing, as experience in attachment prepares one to form a relationship, including that with an idol (Cole and Leets 1999). Moreover, attachment to peers, as facilitated by secure attachment style, contributes to idolizing (Giles and Maltby 2004). In addition, attachment issues with peers facilitate rather than erode idolizing (Moriarty 1992). Secure attachment style can also contribute to idolizing through raising of autonomy (Giles and Maltby 2004; Vivona 2000). Secure attachment style can also contribute to intimacy (Chow et al. 2017; Collins 2002; Miller and Hoicoisitz 2004). In addition, intimacy is a form of idolizing, in terms of romanticizing or befriending (Cole and Leets 1999). Hence, secure attachment style prepares for idolizing through fostering intimacy. Similarly, secure attachment style can facilitate relationships with persons of the opposite sex, which in turn is a predictor of idolizing (Engle and Kasser 2005). Secure attachment style also contributes to trust, which is a basis for idolizing (Boone 2013; Cotterell 1992; Larose and Boivin 1998). In this way, trusting is a general practice facilitated by secure attachment style and conducive to idolizing. Secure attachment style can also erode self-esteem (Sheehan and Noller 2002; Wilkinson 2010). Meanwhile, self-esteem can diminish idolizing (Reeves et al. 2012). Hence, secure attachment style can sustain idolizing through reducing self-esteem. Furthermore, secure attachment style can enhance familiarity with the target of attachment (Monteoliva et al. 2016). Meanwhile, familiarity may be a basis for idolizing (Greene and Adams-Price 1990). Therefore, secure attachment style may prepare for familiarity conducive to idolizing through some generalization of familiarity. In this way, familiarizing can be a generalizable skill or practice.

Idolizing may also influence and thus have positive correlations with secure attachment style, such as when idolizing brings happiness to reinforce secure attachment style (Cohen 2004; La Guardia et al. 2000). Another possibility is that idolizing strengthens friendship making, which in turn reinforces secure attachment style (Allen et al. 2005; Moriarty 1992). More generally, idolizing generalizes the practice of or orientation to liking or attachment, thus reinforcing attachment styles (Sarapin et al. 2015). That is, idolizing provides the opportunity for strengthening attachment and its secure style.

Idolizing of a figure and secure attachment style are also likely to have positive correlations because of the influences of common causes. A source of commonality is the good quality of the target of attachment and idolizing (End et al. 2002; Huang and Mitchell 2014; Ivaldi and O'Neill 2008; Price et al. 2014; Quiroga and Hamilton-Giachritsis 2017; S. Ryu et al. 2007). Such a target tends to be caring, friendly, dedicated, talented, successful, and mentally healthy, and to have some similarity with the youth.

Idolizing of a figure and secure attachment style may maintain a positive correlation because of their impacts on the same consequences. One common consequence is healthy adulthood or personality (Collins 2002; Kroger 1996). On the one hand, idolizing may facilitate learning about talents and other good features from the idol (Greenwood 2007; Sarapin et al. 2015). On the other hand, secure attachment style represents internal working models necessary to social development (Monteoliva et al. 2016). Another common consequence is the number of friends (Mikulincer and Selinger 2001; Moriarty 1992). Accordingly, idolizing may prepare the base for making friends generally (Sarapin et al. 2015). At the same time, secure attachment style can activate sensitivity to others and thus facilitate friend making (Monteoliva et al. 2016).

Negative correlation

Idolizing of a figure is likely to display a negative correlation with secure attachment or a positive correlation with insecure attachment under five conditions: First, the idol and person for attachment or maintaining a relationship are generally or categorically different. Second, secure attachment erodes idolizing. Third, idolizing weakens secure attachment. Fourth, idolizing and secure attachment receive opposite effects from some causes. Fifth, idolizing and secure attachment exert opposite impacts on some consequences.

Idolizing and secure attachment are likely to form a negative correlation because of incongruity between the idol and person for attachment or social interaction generally. Evidently, the idol can be imaginary or fantasized and thus not accessible for attachment or social interaction (Greene and Adams-Price 1990). At best, the idol is for secondary attachment, possibly in a parasocial relationship (Giles and Maltby 2004; Gleason et al. 2017). In addition, the idol can be a nonhuman object (Fetscherin and Barbara 2014; Huang and Mitchell 2014).

Secure attachment may dampen idolizing, thus generating a negative correlation between them. There is evidence for such a dampening effect (Engle and Kasser 2005; Giles and Maltby 2004). Particularly, the effect stems from attachment to parents (Giles and Maltby 2004). Conversely, insecure or anxious-ambivalent attachment underlies idolizing (Cole and Leets 1999).

Idolizing may weaken secure attachment, thus culminating in a negative correlation between them. One possibility is that idolizing raises aggression and criminality, which undercuts the relational basis for secure attachment (Greenwood 2007; Quiroga and Hamilton-Giachritsis 2017; Sheridan et al. 2007). Moreover, idolizing tends to erode satisfaction, which is another basis for reinforcing secure attachment (La Guardia et al. 2000; Scharf and Levy 2015).

Idolizing and secure attachment may maintain a negative correlation due to their divergent responses to some common causes. Notably, the relationship with or availability of parents can strengthen secure attachment but weaken idolizing (Moriarty 1992; Nosko et al. 2011). Moreover, intimacy, relatedness, or popularity as opposed to social isolation can contribute to secure attachment and reduced idolizing (Allen et al. 2005; De Becker et al. 2007; Freeman and Brown 2001; Quiroga and Hamilton-Giachritsis 2017).

Idolizing and secure attachment can also manifest a negative correlation because of their divergent impacts on some common consequences. In terms of well-being, secure attachment can contribute to body satisfaction, whereas idolizing can dampen body satisfaction (Scharf and Levy 2015). In addition, whereas secure attachment can reduce depression, distress, anxiety, fear, loneliness, regret, guilt, and other forms of negative affect, idolizing can elevate these (O. Brown and Symons 2016; Gillath et al. 2005; Hocking et al. 2016; Lavy et al. 2010; Millings et al. 2012; Nishikawa et al. 2010; Permuy et al. 2010; Schimmenti and Bifulco 2015; Wilkinson 2010). Concerning attitudinal consequences, whereas secure attachment can sustain attachment, love, dependence, and trust in people, idolizing can develop loyalty to nonhumans such as the brand and cosmetic surgery (Bidmon 2017; Boone 2013; Bush et al. 2005; Fetscherin and Barbara 2014; Nosko et al. 2011; Swami et al. 2009; Wilkinson 2010). Regarding behavioral consequences, whereas secure attachment can reduce addiction, aggression, argumentativeness, criminality, and other forms of deviance, idolizing can foment them (Greenwood 2007; Grych and Kinsfogel 2010; Y. Jin et al. 2017; Monteoliva et al. 2016; Sheridan et al. 2007). Concerning dispositional consequences, whereas secure attachment can foster prosociality and morality as opposed to private concern, idolizing can impede them (Erez et al. 2008; Moriarty 1992; Walker and Frimer 2009).

Correlations between idolizing and intimacy

A positive correlation between idolizing and intimacy indicates assimilation, expansion, generalizing, or spillover between idolizing and intimacy. That is, when idolizing happens, intimacy also happens and vice versa. By contrast, a negative correlation between idolizing and intimacy reflects contrast, compensating, conflict, or contradiction between idolizing and intimacy. That is, when idolizing is high, intimacy is low and vice versa.

Positive correlation

Idolizing of a figure is likely to maintain a positive correlation with intimacy with the closest friends under five conditions: First, the figure and closest friend have an overlap such that the closest friend is an idol or vice versa. An extreme case is that idolizing and intimacy maintain a part-whole relationship. Essentially, both idolizing and intimacy share a positive valence about social relation. Second, intimacy causes idolizing. Third, idolizing causes intimacy. Fourth, idolizing and intimacy share a common cause. Fifth, idolizing and intimacy have a common consequence.

Idolizing of a figure and intimacy with the closest friend are likely to have a positive correlation because of the overlap between the figure and closest friend and because both idolizing and intimacy share a positive valence. Obviously, the friend can be a figure for idolizing (White and O'Brien 1999). In addition, the friend is a target of attachment, familiarity, intimacy, commitment, and voluntary selection (Meeus et al. 2002; Pellegrini and Blatchford 2000; Rubin et al. 2008; Seibert and Kerns 2009; Wilkinson 2008). The friend also has the features of popularity, influence, and similarity with the youth (Adler and Adler 1998; Bagwell and Schmidt 2011; Espelage et al. 2007; Rose 2002). Similarly, the idol is a target for attachment, familiarity, intimacy, love, and affiliation, including proximity seeking, security, trust, and romance (Cole and Leets 1999; Cotterell 1992; de Jong 1992; Ellison 1991; Fetscherin and Barbara 2014; Greene and Adams-Price 1990; Hafner 2009; Larose and Boivin 1998). Moreover, the idol is a target for emulation, modeling, and limitation, thus leading to similarity between the idol and its worshipper (Bowers et al. 2016; Raviv et al. 1996; Robinson et al. 2016; C. Wang et al. 2009). The idol is also influential such as on consumption, commitment, and obsession (Lindenberg et al. 2011; McCutchson et al. 2002; C. Wang et al. 2009). Furthermore, the idol is likely to have the credits of popularity, sociability, and prestige (Holub et al. 2008; Robinson et al. 2016). Obviously, the idol can be a target for intimacy (Boon and Lomore 2001; Greenwood and Long 2011; S. Johnson et al. 2016). Essentially, intimacy has such positive valences as competence, complementarity to life, and nondeviance or normalcy (K. Chou 2000; Greenwood and Long 2011; Henderson et al. 2009). Meanwhile, idolizing has such positive or desirable features as attachment or security, catharsis, entertainment, playing, normalcy, identity construction, self-concept development, and being functional to the person (Adams-Price and Greene 1990; Giles 2000; Karniol 2001; Lin and Lin 2007; Madhavan and Crowell 2014; Maltby et al. 2006; McCutcheon et al. 2003; Pleiss and Feldhusen 1995; Raviv et al. 1996; Stevens 2010). Moreover, idolizing can contribute to social integration (Turner and Scherman 1996).

Idolizing of a figure is also likely to be a consequence of intimacy with the closest friends, thus buttressing their positive correlation. The simplest case is that idolizing of a figure such as a stranger is a generalization of intimacy with the closest friend (Ferris 2001; Stevens 2010). Essentially, intimacy with or romanticizing the idol is a form of idolizing (Cole and Leets 1999). Moreover commodifying the idol is a way of fabricating intimacy with the idol (Schultze et al. 1991). Idolizing in terms of attachment is also a form of intimacy (Ellison 1991). More generally, intimacy indicators that induce idolizing include attachment to peers, having parents, and having no peer conflict (Giles and Maltby 2004; Moriarty 1992). Essentially, secure attachment rather than anxious, avoidant, or hostile attachment is crucial to explain the positive impact of the intimacy of idolizing (Cole and Leets 1999). In·this regard, secure attachment, primarily resting on the caretaker's responsiveness during young childhood, shapes attachment and intimacy throughout life. Furthermore, intimacy can contribute to relational competence, sensitivity, and trust (Henderson et al. 2009). These qualities tend to underlie idolizing (Cotterell 1992; Engle and Kasser 2005; Larose and Boivin 1998). Moreover, intimacy maintained through dating can contribute to idolizing, probably reflecting an extension from the dating partner to the idol (Engle and Kasser 2005). An obvious explanation is that intimacy reflects attachment security, which is contributory to idolizing (Cole and Leats 1999).

Idolizing of a figure and intimacy with the closest friends are also likely to maintain a correlation because of the effect of idolizing on intimacy. Accordingly, idolizing can facilitate friendship making (Moriarty 1992). One possibility is that idolizing activates friendship making to generalize from the idol to others (Giles and Malltby 2004; Gleason et al. 2017). Another possibility is that idolizing fosters social activities such as those with a fan club to facilitate friendship making (Turner and Scherman 1996). In addition, idolizing may have a prosocial tendency to uphold friendship making (Calvert et al. 2004). Such friendship making practice or orientation tends to foster intimacy (Bauminger et al. 2008; Collins 2002). Moreover, friends are helpful in strengthening intimacy with others (Eyal and Dailey 2012). An explanation is that idolizing reflects social cohesion, which bolsters intimacy (Georgas et al. 1997). That is, friendliness or supportiveness toward the idol and others facilitates intimacy.

The positive correlation between idolizing of a figure and intimacy with the closest friend is also likely to arise from influences from common causes. Common attitudinal causes appear to be attachment, identification, or commitment to social relations or peers (Eyal and Dailey 2012; Giles and Maltby 2004). Moreover, the trait of nonavoidance in attachment is a common cause (Chow et al. 2017; Collins 2002). In addition, common background causes appear to be age and female gender (Eyal and Dailey 2012; Lempers and Clark-Lempers 1993; Giles and Maltby 2004). The age effect reflects the influence of pubertal development and other forms of maturation (Greene and Adams-Price 1990). Meanwhile, the gender effect reflects the sociobiological difference (Henry 1983). An explanation is that both intimacy and idolizing arise from the need for sex and reproduction associated with maturation (Giles 2000; Rusch et al. 2015).

The positive correlation between idolizing of a figure and intimacy may also be because of their common consequences. One common consequence has been friendship making or strengthening or social enhancement (Hand et al. 2013; Henderson et al. 2009; Moriarty 1992). Accordingly, social enhancement may stem from attachment security underlying both intimacy and idolizing (Arseth et al. 2009; Cole and Leets 1999). Thus, attachment security developed in early life can buttress exploration to enhance both idolizing and intimacy.

Negative correlation

Idolizing of a figure is likely to hold a negative correlation with intimacy with the closest friend under five conditions: First, the idol and friend are categorically different. Second, intimacy with the closest friend impedes idolizing. Third, idolizing impairs intimacy. Fourth, idolizing and intimacy receive opposite effects from some causes. Fifth, idolizing and intimacy exert opposite influences on some consequences.

Idolizing of a figure and intimacy with the closest friend are likely to maintain a negative correlation because of a discrepancy between the idol and friend. Obviously, whereas the closest friend tends to manifest mutuality or reciprocity, an idol other than a friend cannot have this property (Bagwell and Schmidt 2011; Greene and Adams-Price 1990; Scholte et al. 2009). Notably, the closest friend rather than the idol would be involved in conversation (Morgan and Korobov 2012). Meanwhile, the idol can be imagined, fantasized, or parasocial, whereas the closest friend would be a real person (Cole and Leets 1999; J. Turner 1993).

Intimacy with the closest friend is likely to exert a negative effect on idolizing, thus manifesting a negative correlation between intimacy and idolizing. For instance, conflict with the friend, which reflects inadequate intimacy with the friend, supports idolizing (Moriarty 1992). Moreover, intimacy sustains satisfaction, which in turn dampens idolizing (Hand et al. 2013; Reeves et al. 2012). In addition, intimacy enhances self-efficacy, which diminishes idolizing (Henderson et al. 2009; Reeves et al. 2012). An explanation for the effect of intimacy is its erosion of empty self, which underlies idolizing (Reeves et al. 2012).

Idolizing of a figure is also likely to impede intimacy with the closest friend, hence exhibiting a negative correlation between idolizing and intimacy. Notably, idolizing fosters the need for privacy, which may impede intimacy with friends, such as through the need for belonging (Greenwood and Long 2011; Moriarty 1992). Moreover, idolizing can foment aggression, which reflects dysregulation, which in turn impairs intimacy (Greenwood 2007; Roth and Assor 2012). In addition, idolizing can foment maladjustment and feelings of guilt, which represent negative affect, impeding intimacy (Julal et al. 2017; Moriarty 1992; Scharf and Levy 2015). An obvious explanation is that intimacy with the closest friend displaces the social or parasocial need for an idol (Eyal and Dailey 2012).

Idolizing and intimacy are likely to manifest a negative correlation because of their divergent responses to some common causes. Causes such as boredom and negative affect generally raise idolizing but attenuate intimacy (Julal et al. 2017; Reeves et al. 2012). Moreover, attachment security as opposed to anxiety and avoidance sustains intimacy but impedes idolizing (Bauminger et al. 2009; Chow et al. 2017; Collins 2002; Miller and Hoicoisitz 2004; Giles and Maltby 2004). Whereas Internet or online use, as a behavioral cause, facilitates idolizing, it impedes intimacy (Earl and Kimport 2009; Hand et al. 2013; Y. Huang 2006). In terms of experience, whereas approval from the social network or peers is conducive to intimacy, it tends to impede idolizing (Eyal and Dailey 2012; Moriarty 1992). Regarding the cause of need, whereas need for belonging sustains intimacy, need for power underlies idolizing (Greenwood and Long 2011; Moriarty 1992).

Idolizing and intimacy are also likely to display a negative correlation because of their divergent impacts or consequences. Regarding well-being, whereas intimacy buttresses satisfaction, idolizing impairs it (Hand et al. 2013;

Scharf and Levy 2015). In addition, whereas intimacy prevents negative affect, idolizing foments it (Arseth et al. 2009; Moriarty 1992; Scharf and Levy 2015). Concerning behavioral outcomes, whereas intimacy reduces deviance, doping, and/or criminality, idolizing foments them (K. Chou 2000; Shadur and Hussong 2014; Sheridan et al. 2007). In terms of skill, whereas intimacy supports competence, idolizing hinders it (Houran et al. 2005).

Correlation between idolizing and star worship

Stars in entertainment, sports, and other fields are more likely than others to be the target for idolizing, encompassing glorifying, idealizing, beautifying, crediting, glamourizing, prizing, commodifying, faming, romanticizing, befriending, popularizing, and personalizing. Essentially, stars treasure and capitalize on the qualities for idolizing, including glory, beauty, merit, glamour, marketability, fame, romance, friendliness, popularity, and availability for choice (Argyle 1994; De Backer 2012; Lin and Lin 2007). Idolizing is therefore likely to apply to stars and have a positive correlation with star worship.

Background influences

Background characteristics, including age, sex, education, parental education, the region (i.e., Hong Kong vs. Mainland China), and fan club membership, can influence idolizing and/or related concerns about the spillover or compensation of idolizing. Whereas the spillover or assimilation thesis suggests that idolizing has positive correlations with self-efficacy, secure attachment, and intimacy, the compensation or contrast thesis envisions negative correlations between idolizing and the latter.

Age effects on idolizing

Relevant to the understanding of the negative effect of age on idolizing is the consideration that idolizing results from immature or inadequate development in cognitive and psychic or psychoanalytic aspects. Accordingly, egocentrism, imaginativeness, and fabling as immature cognitive development as opposed to realistic deliberation are responsible for idolizing (Seiffge-Krenke 1997). Thus, cognitive deficit and inflexibility engender idolizing (Maltby et al. 2004; McCutcheon et al. 2003). Conversely, creativity, critical thinking, crystallized intelligence, spatial ability, and need for cognition, which register cognitive competence, prevent idolizing. Furthermore, inadequate psychic or ego development signified by narcissism, pursuit of freedom, projection of wishes, fear of separation, and expression of sexual instinct tends to underlie idolizing (Driscoll 1999; Giles 2000; Noser and Zeigler-Hill 2014; Seiffge-Krenke 1997). That is, impulsivity and agitation as opposed to self-control, adjustment, and socialization or cultivation breed idolizing. Such inadequate development can result from attachment problems or irresponsive caretaking received, which foments attachment anxiety or jealousy (Cole and Leets 1999). That is, when the caretaker is unavailable, unresponsive, and not trustworthy, anxiety concerning attachment and separation grow to propel idolizing. The inadequate development also compromises the youth's identity, and this effect is a possible determinant of idolizing (Maltby et al. 2004b; McCutcheon et al. 2003). Similarly, a fragile self can be a cause of idolizing (Jenson 1992; Reeves et al. 2012). Moreover, depression, isolation, and lack of alliances and community are likely to precede idolizing (Jenson 1992; Reeves et al. 2012). Essentially, inadequate or immature development in cognitive and psychic aspects obviously diminishes with aging (Brouwers et al. 2006; Gormley et al. 2005; Thompson and Norris 1982; Tinsley and Spencer 2010).

The older youth mainly displays less idolizing (Raviv et al. 1996; Sivami et al. 2010; C. Wang et al. 2009). Particularly, the post-adolescent youth idolizes less than does the adolescent (Gleason et al. 2017). The lower level of idolizing in the older youth may be attributable to identity and cognitive development and involvement in community that come with age (Reeves et al. 2012; Seiffge-Krenke 1997). Clearly, education, identity achievement, cognitive development, moral development, critical thinking, and community service increase with age (Kramer and Melchoir 1990; Markoulis and Valanides 1997; Niemi and Klingler 2012; Pinquart and Pfeiffer 2013; Sanchirico 1991; Wires et al. 1994). Notably, cognitive deficit and rigid thinking precede idolizing, whereas cognitive flexibility and complexity weaken idolizing (Maltby et al. 2004; McCutcheon et al. 2003; Moriarty 1992). Age is essentially an indicator or proxy for cognitive development (Owens et al. 2005). Hence, when the youth is more educated, autonomous, thoughtful, established psychologically, and involved socially, he or she is less demanding on the idol to find support or emulation. Similarly, the older youth is better adjusted and adapted, committed to career, friendship, intimacy, and mobilizing social support (Bokhorst et al. 2009; Jing et al. 1995; O'Connor et al. 2004; Pinquart and Pfeiffer 2013; Zimmer-Gembeck et al. 2012). Such developmental characteristics, involving satisfaction, social security, and occupational status, are likely to dampen idolizing (Argyle 1994; Giles and Maltby 2004; Reeves et al. 2012). In addition, the older youth manifests lower anxiety or fear, distress, identity diffusion, and family strain (Attar-Schwartz et al. 2009; Grasmick et al. 1996; Hay 2003; Ickes et al. 2012; Lorant and Nicaise 2015; Rosenfield et al. 2005; Springer et al. 2007; Thompson and Norris 1992). Behaviorally, the older youth exhibits lower normlessness, Internet use, risk preference, alcoholism, misbehavior, school dropout, delinquency, disruptiveness, doping, theft, violence, and recidivism (Crosnoe and Elder 2004; Jang and Franzen 2013; Mesch 2001; Peltonen et al. 2010; Perron and Howard 2008; Reio et al. 2009; Reynolds and Crea 2015; Vitaro et al. 2005; Wexler et al. 1990). The older youth also has fewer experiences of social rejection, victimization, and psychopathology (Bouchard et al. 2012; Dorahy et al. 2003; van Lier et al. 2005). These features tend to sustain idolizing in view of its prediction by boredom, Internet use, peer conflict, threat received, and psychopathy (Earl and Kimport 2009; Moriarty 1992; Reeves et al. 2012; Southard and Zeigler-Hill 2016).

The older youth is more likely to manifest compensation rather than spillover with idolizing, self-efficacy, attachment, and intimacy, considering his or her greater cognitive development. Essentially, growing in age is a definite indicator of growing in cognitive development (Owens et al. 2005). Moreover, cognitive development means advancement in awareness, differentiation, diversification, and exchange (Bradley et al. 1988; Harter 2012; LeMare and Rubin 1987). That is, cognitive development raises awareness about difference and compensation through exchange. These features are bases for setting boundaries integral to compensation (Greenwood and Long 2011). Hence, increased compensation with age has happened in the negative effect of poor self-feeling on theft (Regnerus 2002). Accordingly, the older youth is more likely to commit theft to compensate for a poor feeling about self. Similarly, increased compensation has happened in effect of the unavailability of friends on theft (Regnerus 2002). That is, the older youth has greater compensation for the unavailability of his or her friends. The effect of compensation has been negative in terms of family communication and attendance at social service programs. Thus, the older youth has greater program attendance as compensation for inadequate family communication. Similarly, the older youth has greater association with a gang as compensation for his or her parents' secrecy or unavailability (Glatz and Dahl 2014). Using doping to compensate for parents' lack of warmth also occurs in the older youth (Pires and Jenkins 2007). Likewise, doping is a more likely compensation for lack of partnership in the older youth (Schulenberg et al. 2000). Association with delinquent peers as compensation for detachment from school is also greater in the older youth (Jang 1999). Conversely, age diminishes spillover in prosociality. Thus, the association between prosocial reasoning and prosocial motivation is weaker in the older youth (Janssens and Dekovic 1997). Moreover, association between one's own smoking and friends' smoking is weaker in the older youth (Stanton et al. 1996). Similarly, the older youth shows a weaker association between his or her doping and peers' doping (Simons-Morton and Chen 2006). Furthermore, the effect of receiving social rejection on doping is weaker in the older youth (Pires and Jenkins 2007). That is, spillover from the adverse experience of social rejection to the adverse behavior of doping is weaker in the older youth. Similarly, spillover from the experience of victimization to delinquency is weaker in the older youth (Benda and Corwyn 2002).

Gender effects on idolizing

Gender makes a difference in idolizing primarily through evolutionary, psychoanalytic, and sociocultural mechanisms. Accordingly, gender differences arise due to these mechanisms (Aslan 2015; Dunkel et al. 2016; Galambos et al. 2009; Sumter et al. 2013; Zupancic et al. 2014). Meanwhile, idolizing is a function of the same mechanisms (De Backer et al. 2007; Giles 2000; Noser and Zeigler-Hill 2014; Robinson et al. 2016; Seiffge-Krenke 1997). Considering the mechanisms, the girl is likely to manifest greater idolizing than is the boy. This happens, according to the evolutionary mechanism, as the girl is more predisposed to childcare and its necessary dependence on help through association and affiliation with resourceful people than is the boy (Dunkel et al. 2016; Galambos et al. 2009). Essentially, these differences have evolved through millennia and have been genetically entrenched in youth. Consistent with the evolutionary mechanism is the psychoanalytic mechanism, which highlights the girl's need for security due to her sexual energy and intuition (Aslan 2015). Hence, seeking affiliation and support characterizes the girl. These mechanisms also benefit from reinforcement through the sociocultural mechanism, which buttresses the girl's higher dependence, relationship maintenance, and emotional expression, particularly in the absence of actual sexual activity, more so than the boy's (Sumter et al. 2013; Zupancic et al. 2014). These mechanisms commonly lead to the girl's greater attachment to parents and the romantic partner (Adams-Price and Greene 1990; Argyle 1994; Bellair and Roscigno 2000; Greene and Adams-Price 1990). In this connection, the girl favors romance rather than realistic contact more so than the boy (Feiring 1995). Similarly, the girl is also more likely to have group membership than the boy (Newman et al. 2007). Behaviorally, the girl has more dating, romantic, conforming, recourse, and pop music involvement than the boy (Cavanagh 2007; Cornell et al. 2014; Feiring 1995; Furman and Winkles 2010; Frith 1983; Gonzalez et al. 2016; McCarthy and Casey 2008; Wilder et al. 2000; Zupancic et al. 2014). In contrast, the girl has lower sexual engagement than the boy (Cavanagh 2007; Dorius et al. 1993). Accordingly, the girl prefers affective and romantic engagements to sexual ones. Eventually, the girl has the traits of dependability, sensitivity, and susceptibility to others (Hill and Rojewski 1999; Unger et al. 2001; Weems et al. 2002). With these traits, the girl exhibits such states or feelings of intimacy and love more than the boy (Lempers and Clark-Lempers 1993; Ross and Mirowsky 1989; Shimai et al. 2006; Sumter et al. 2013). Conversely, the girl displays lower self-esteem than the boy (Bjarnason 2009; Broh 2002; Fredricks and Eccles 2005; Lessard et al. 2011; Wilkinson 2010; Wouters et al. 2013). Therefore, the girl displays greater romantic idolizing than the boy (Adams-Price and Greene 1990; He and Feng 2002; S. Ryu et al. 2007; Sivami et al. 2010). These attitudes, behaviors, traits, and feelings are responsible for idolizing. Notably, the attitude of attachment to peers sustains idolizing (Giles and Maltby 2004). The behaviors of dating, daydreaming, pop music involvement, and parasocial interaction rather than realistic interaction underlie idolizing (Cole and Leets 1999; Engle and Kasser 2005; Moriarty 1992; Seiffge-Krenke 1997). The feeling of self-esteem diminishes idolizing, meaning that the youth with lower self-esteem has higher idolizing (Reeves et al. 2012).

The girl is likely to show more compensation or contrast and less spillover or generalization than is the boy. This gender difference also has evolutionary, psychoanalytic, and sociocultural bases. The evolutionary perspective holds that the girl is more concerned than is the boy about childcare or its preparation, thus requiring security through carefulness, selectivity, and differentiation (Dunkel et al. 2016; Galambos et al. 2009). Such characteristics sustain compensation (Cambon et al. 2015). From the psychoanalytic perspective, the girl has greater feelings of insecurity, inferiority, and deficit stemming from sexual characteristics than does the boy, meaning she has greater need for compensation (Dacey and Lennon 1998; Granquist and Dickie 2005; King and Roeser 2009; Seiffge-Krenke 1997). From the sociocultural perspective, moreover, the girl learns to emphasize attachment, involvement, and intimacy more so than does the boy to sustain the need for compensation rather than spillover, particularly concerning attachment, involvement, and intimacy (East 2009; Zupancic et al. 2014).

Spillover is weaker in the girl than in the boy in the following ways. Most obviously, the girl manifests weaker stability in depression, doping, and friendship quality (Brensilver et al. 2011; Mayet et al. 2012; Prinstein et al. 2005). Moreover, spillover is lower in the girl than in the boy in the contributions of social anxiety to depression (Prinstein 2007). Similarly, the girl shows a lower contribution of self-discrepancy to depression than does the boy (Alfeld-Liro and Sigelman 1998). Moreover, the contributions of antipathy to depression and violence are lower in the girl than in the boy (Schwartz et al. 2003). Another instance of lower spillover is the lower contribution of strain to delinquency in the girl than in the boy (Hay 2003). The lower contribution of academic achievement to family functioning in the girl than in the boy also represents weaker spillover in the girl (Chui and Wong 2017). Furthermore, aggression displays lower contributions to alcoholism, smoking, doping, and distress, suggesting lower spillover from aggression to other problems (Flannery et al. 1993; Piko et al. 2006).

In addition, the contribution of delinquency to depression is lower in the girl than in the boy (Connell and Dishion 2006). Another instance of lower spillover is the weaker contribution of doping to alcoholism in the girl than in the boy (Light et al. 2003). Likewise, the contribution of externalizing to depression is weaker in the girl than in the boy (Wiesner and Kim 2006). Clearly, spillover is lower in the girl than in the boy in terms of the contribution of pornography use to rape. That is, the girl's use of pornography is less likely to foment rape than is the boy's use. Furthermore, the contribution of withdrawal to social disintegration is weaker in the girl than in the boy (Valdivia et al. 2005). The experience of control or protection shows a weaker effect on preventing delinquency in the girl than in the boy (Jessor et al. 2003). This is another instance of weaker spillover in the girl. Similarly, the contribution of parental disapproval of alcoholism to preventing alcoholism is weaker in the girl than in the boy (Kelly et al. 2011). Furthermore, the contribution of the norm of doping among peers to doping is weaker in the girl than in the boy (Callas et al. 2004). An obvious weaker instance of spillover in the girl than in the boy is also evident in the contribution of perceived environmental problems to endorsement for environmentalism (K. Lee 2009). Furthermore, programs for enhancing social competence are less effective to the girl than to the boy (Liang et al. 2008). Self-efficacy in volunteering also contributes less to volunteering in the girl than in the boy (Lindenmeier 2008). Conversely, the contributions of self-control including impulsivity and preference for simplicity in work to theft are weaker in the girl than in the boy (Chui and Chan 2016). Lower spillover in the girl than in the boy is also evident in the contribution of parental substance use to delinquency (Storvoll and Wichstrom 2002). A clear instance of weaker spillover in the girl than in the boy is also evident in the contribution of friends' smoking to one's own smoking (Crosnoe et al. 2002). Similarly, the contributions of unemployment in the community and peers to one's own unemployment is weaker in the girl than in the boy (Aberg and Hedstrom 2011).

Compensation or contrast is greater in the girl than in the boy. Such a gender difference is the negative effect of attachment to adults and interaction with parents on delinquency, suggesting a displacement of delinquency (Griffin et al. 2000; Huebner and Betts 2002). Delinquency is also a greater displacement of depression in the girl than in the boy (Connell and Dishion 2006). Another gender difference in displacement by activity, including dating, is evident in academic achievement (Giordano et al. 2008; Holland and Andre 1987; Huebner and Betts 2002). In contrast, the displacement of externalizing behavior by organized activity and school performance is greater in the girl than in the boy (Storvoll and Wichstrom 2002). At the same time, externalizing behavior shows a greater displacement of depression in the girl than in the boy (Wiesner and Kim 2006). The girl also displays a greater displacement in resilience by avoidant coping (Markstrom et al. 2000). Furthermore, sport or athletic participation displaces sexual activity more intensely in the girl than in the boy (Miller et al. 1986). Hence, the girl exhibits greater behavioral compensation or displacement than does the boy.

Region effects on idolizing

The Mainland Chinese youth is likely to exhibit greater idolizing than his or her counterpart in Hong Kong. Evidently, idolizing or idolatry is popular in Mainland China (Clark 2012). As such, admiring, esteem, respecting, yearning for, envying, revering, adoring, and being addicted to idols is widespread there (He 2006). Particularly, pop stars there are the common target for idolizing or worshipping (Qi and Tang 2004). This phenomenon may rest on the cultural bases of collectivism, Confucianism, obedience, compliance, deference, respect, and normativity, which are salient in Mainland China (Cheung and Pomerantz 2011; Liao et al. 2011; C. Liu et al. 2005; Peng et al. 2015; Zhan and Ning 2004; Zhang 2003). These cultural bases encourage respecting, obeying, adoring, conforming to, and compliance with idols in order to locate and follow norms (Bush et al. 2002; Nelson and Barry 2005; Peng et al. 2015; Zhou et al. 2004). Another significant basis is the political one, particularly through education, including moral, civic, character, patriotic, and political education (Jiang et al. 1993; Lawrence 2000; Wu 2003). Such political or educational force encourages idolatry or modeling of patriotic and other successful and exalted heroes.

Conversely, the youth in Hong Kong is less likely to show idolizing than is his or her counterpart in Mainland China. The cultural account suggests that the youth in Hong Kong is low in conventionality and trust in authority (H. Ng 2015). These characteristics discourage idolizing and modeling to learn conventions or norms. Another cultural basis is religion, which is more influential in Hong Kong than in Mainland China (King and Roeser 2009; Nelson and Barry 2005; Zhang and Thomas 1994). The religious influence discourages idolizing, especially of nonreligious figures. This restricts idolizing, as most idols are nonreligious figures. An alternative account is that idols are just too common in Hong Kong such that their value for idolizing depreciates there (Lee and Ting 2015). That is, when idols are rare and selected, they are worthy of idolizing. The ubiquity of idols in Hong Kong is attributable to the boost of the entertainment industry to consolidate consumerism (Irazabal and Chakravarty 2007). Hence, the quantity of idols reduces their quality and therefore value for admiration or idolizing. Furthermore, the youth in Hong Kong shows lower curiosity than does the youth elsewhere (Fairbrother 2003). This may weaken the youth's idolizing as a way to fulfill curiosity.

The youth in Hong Kong is also more likely to display compensation rather than spillover than is the Mainland Chinese youth. Culturally, compensation reflects differentiation, calculation, resistance, and antagonism rather than tolerance, submission, and compliance, which are salient in Hong Kong (Lam et al. 2001; F. Lee et al. 2017; Tse 2007). Conversely, the ethos salient in Mainland China emphasizes adjustment, forbearance, compliance, conformity, and obedience (Cui et al. 2016; Liao et al. 2011; Liu et al. 2005; Zhan and Ning 2004; Zhang 2003; Zhu 2006). As such, the Mainland Chinese youth shows lower confrontation than does the other (Keller and Loewenstein 2011). Conversely, the former is fonder of the maintenance of synthesis, harmony, balance, and compromise than is the other (Peng and Nisbett 1999; Spencer-Rodgers et al. 2010). The Mainland Chinese youth is also less active and assertive than the other (Heffernan et al. 2010; Keller and Loewenstein 2011). Conversely, the former is more friendly and compliant (Keller and Loewenstein 2011; Zhang and Thomas 1994). These qualities are likely to buttress spillover or assimilation as opposed to compensation or contrast. They also echo the corresponding cultural ethos highlighting conformity, compliance, and obedience in Mainland China (Bush et al. 2002; Cui et al. 2016; Liao et al. 2011; Liu et al. 2006; Nelson and Barry 2005; Peng et al. 2015; Zhou et al. 2004; Zhu 2006).

Education effects on idolizing

Education is likely to lower idolizing such that idolizing reduces as the child moves up in school grade. The casual logic, similar to that of age, represents cognitive development or cognitive apprenticeship (Furnham-Diggory 1992). According to this logic, education teaches and enhances knowledge and strategies or heuristics of learning, control, and problem solving. Education proceeds through and thereby exemplifies and strengthens verbalization, articulation, exploration, modeling, reflection, and scaffolding, which supports learning. Moreover, education induces cognitive development sequentially with increasing diversity, complexity, and specification. What is more, education facilitates social development in cooperation, intrinsic motivation, expert culture, and situated learning, which is a generalization of learning to any situation encountered. In all, cognitive development through education sharpens, extols, and sanctifies personal capability and expertise. Meanwhile, cognitive development diminishes idolizing with a reduction in egocentrism, which upholds imagination rather than learning (Seiffge-Krenke 1997). That is, education fosters learning capacity and spirit to erode unrealistic expectations and projection through idolizing.

In line with the logic of cognitive development, education shows direct and indirect negative impacts on idolizing. Accordingly, idolizing is lower with higher education (Hoegele et al. 2014). Moreover, education incubates the traits of creativity, cognitive complexity, curiosity, internal control, and scientific knowledge (Bidwell et al. 1996; Crystal and DeBell 2002; Moneta et al. 2001; Simonton 1981, 1994; C. Yi et al. 2004). These traits, notably cognitive complexity, dampen idolizing (Maltby et al. 2004; Moriarty 1992). Conversely, education reduces the values of fatalism, hedonism, and romanticism (Bynner and Parsons 2002; Eggermant 2004; Thompson and Norris 1992; Verhagen et al. 2000). These values or orientations, involving materialism, grandiosity, and rigid thinking, tend to underlie idolizing (Maltby et al. 2006; Moriarty 1992; Southard and Zeigler-Hill 2016). Education also increases favor for education, career motivation, occupational aspiration, and work ethics (Lowe and Krahn 2000; Moore and Keith 1992; Watson et al. 2002). Such developmental orientations tend to be at odds with idolizing (Gleason et al. 2017). Behaviorally, education propels volunteering, community participation, financial activity, job search, life planning, and political engagement and participation (Danes et al. 2013; Fahmy 2006; Hellevik and Steersten 2013; Kim and Wilcox 2013; Koh et al. 2013; Mandell and Klein 2009; Marks 2005; Matthews and Howell 2006; Niemi et al. 2000). Such activities are disparate from homebound activities such as television watching, music listening, Internet use, parasocial interaction, and even daydreaming, which precipitates idolizing (Cole and Leets 1999; De Backer et al. 2007; Earl and Kimport 2009; Moriarty 1992; Price et al. 2014; J. Turner 1993; Seiffge-Krenke 1997). In addition, education reduces family time and home chores (Helwig 2004; Larson and Richards 1991). Furthermore, education buttresses adjustment, self-efficacy, and mastery (Liu and Chen 2010; Rawlings 2012; Ross and Mirowsky 1989). These conditions impede idolizing (Giles and Maltby 2004; Reeves et al. 2012).

Parental education effects on idolizing

Parental education is also likely to attenuate the youth's idolizing. Such education is a resource to the youth, thus helping the youth accomplish various tasks (Almgren et al. 2009; Steele et al. 2005). The accomplishment can be evident in the youth's academic achievement and intellectual development (Gormley et al. 2005; Lauglo 2011; Pong et al. 2010). Hence, the youth's cognitive development again benefits from parental education. Such development is likely to diminish idolizing. Evidently, parental education cultivates the youth's traits of critical thinking and internal control (Dehejia et al. 2009; Terenzini et al. 1993). Such cognitive traits dampen idolizing (McCutcheon et al. 2003). Parental education also enhances the youth's attachment and closeness to parents (Campbell and Eggerling-Boeck 2006; Diener et al. 2003). The attachment erodes idolizing (Giles and Maltby 2004). Conversely, parental education reduces the youth's political interest (Ekstrom and Ostman 2013). This interest contributes to idolizing (S. Ryu et al. 2007). Moreover, parental education reduces the youth's illness and relational stress, problems, and risk (Axinn et al. 1999; Charles et al. 2004; Springer et al. 2007; Woodward and Fergusson 1999). These problems breed idolizing (Moriarty 1992). Regarding well-being, parental education stabilizes the youth's adjustment, satisfaction, self-efficacy, self-esteem, development, health, and social integration (Azfredrick 2015; Benson et al. 2011; Broh 2002; Gibson 2001; Hansell and White 1991; Hirschi 2009; Hickman et al. 2000; Mortimer 2003; Rose-Krasnor et al. 2005). At the same time, such well-being diminishes idolizing (Reeves et al. 2012). In addition, parental education prevents the youth's depression and family strain (Hagan and Foster 2001; Hay 2003; Mortimer et al. 2002). Such ill-being engenders idolizing (Reeves et al. 2012). Hence, parental education is likely to attenuate the youth's idolizing at least indirectly.

Fan club membership effects on idolizing

Fan club membership is likely to boost idolizing. Such membership, by nature, is a form of collective commitment to a particular recreation or interest. It thus gathers social capital to facilitate actions (Martin 2009). Essentially, membership in any club functions to draw social and thereby other socially mediated resources to heighten capability and then raise motivation. That is, membership performs the chief function of activation or potentiating. Club membership thereby enhances such attitudes as aspiration, attachment, and interest, particularly those compatible with the club (Martin 2009; Fredricks and Eccles 2005; Rose-Krasnor et al. 2005). Behaviorally, club membership uplifts engagement, working, and achievement, such as those in school and volunteering (Cruce and Moore 2007; Dumais 2006; Eccles and Barber 1999; Fredricks and Eccles 2005; Marks and Jones 2004; McLellan and Youniss 2003). Meanwhile, gang membership activates delinquency, including prostitution and violence (Agnew 2002; Broidy 2001; Cusick 2002; Jessor et al. 2003; Rose-Krasnor et al. 2005; Vowell and May 2000; Wright and Fitzpatrick 2006). Plausibly, membership provides esoteric resources to enable actions, particularly those congenial with the membership. Membership in a fan club is thereby likely to heighten idolizing of the idol adored in the club.

Summary

Idolatry comprises choosing and accepting an idol for idolizing. The idol can be a celebrity, luminary, entertainer, star, hero, family member, teacher, fictional figure, or historical character. Idolizing, predicated on the functionalist conceptualization, comprises 11 primary or first-order components to demonstrate the four requisite functions of fulfillment, adaptation, integration, and latency for any action. That is, the components need to fulfill the goal, adapt to the environment, integrate elements, and maintain or perpetuate the pattern in the action, such as idolizing. The 11 primary components are idealizing, beautifying, crediting, glamourizing, and modeling for the primary function of fulfillment;

commodifying and faming for the primary function of adaptation; romanticizing, befriending, and popularizing for the primary function of integration; and personalizing for the primary function of latency. Furthermore, glamourizing, beautifying, faming, and crediting represent the second-order component of glorifying, whereas commodifying, idealizing, befriending, and romanticizing register the second-order component of prizing.

It is possible for idolatry to maintain positive or negative relationships with self-efficacy belief, secure attachment style, and intimacy. Whereas the positive relationships uphold the spillover thesis about generalization, extension, and/or assimilation between idolatry and other engagements, the negative relationships buttress the compensation about displacement, competition, and/or contrast between idolatry and others. The spillover thesis is obviously plausible because of overlap between the idol and actual or ideal self, closest friends, and other people generally. Moreover, the spillover is explicable with the mechanisms of attachment, social cohesion, maturation and thus social or sexual need, social learning, and formation of personal and social identity. That is, these mechanisms underlie idolizing, self-efficacy, attachment, and/or intimacy. By contrast, the compensation thesis rests on notions of empty self, displacement, social comparison, and threat. As such, idolizing and other engagements are competing among themselves. The plausibility of the apparent contradictory theses of spillover and compensation indicates the need for empirical examination to resolve the contradiction.

Idolizing and compensation versus spillover are also plausible susceptible to age, gender, and the region in China, the Mainland versus Hong Kong. Age or education also indicates that cognitive development, which erodes egocentrism, is likely to reduce idolizing and spillover. Females, due to evolutionary reasons, are likely to idolize selectively, thus upholding compensation rather than spillover. Mainland Chinese youth, because of their traditional and nationalist or patriotic culture, are fond of idolizing or modeling in a generalizing way consistent with the spillover thesis. In contrast, Hong Kong youth are likely to be selective in idolizing, probably because of availability of competitive idols, especially marketed by the entertainment industry. Hence, idolizing and its spillover are likely to be lower in Hong Kong than in Mainland China.

Part 2: New findings in China

The issue concerning compensation and spillover among idolatry and other relationships is a focus of empirical inquiry in China, involving both Hong Kong and Mainland Chinese. Herein, the compensation thesis holds that idolatry and other relationships are compensatory or replaceable with each other (Argyle 1994; Engle and Kasser 2005; Feldman and Wentzel 1995; Jenson 1992). The compensation thus suggests that deficiency in relationship or engagement with one or another prompts idolatry. By contrast, the spillover thesis maintains that idolatry and other engagements extend, enhance, or generalize to each other (Engle and Kasser 2005). The concept of spillover therefore means that idolatry results from another engagement or vice versa. More specifically, the compensation thesis posits negative relationships between idolatry and other engagements such as self-efficacy, secure attachment, and intimacy with the closest friend. On the contrary, the spillover thesis posits positive relationships between idolatry and engagements. Clarifying compensation and spillover in idolatry is vital to determine the origins and consequences of idolatry. To be good, idolatry would exhibit spillover such that it has a basis or consequence in other good engagements such as self-efficacy, secure attachment, and intimacy. Conversely, idolatry is undesirable when it manifests compensation or displacement with favorable engagements. Such assessment of goodness is justifiable with all the consequentialist, teleological, utilitarian, and deontological or formalist principles. Accordingly, whether idolatry is good or bad depends on its bases and/or consequences (Aquino and Freeman 2009; Hamilton 2010; Richmond and Cummings 2004). Thus, self-efficacy, attachment security, and intimacy are both extrinsically and intrinsically good (Cotterell 2007; Fosco and Feinberg 2015; Hand et al. 2013; Henderson et al. 2009; Hirschi 2009; Vivona 2000).

Data came from a survey of 1,641 secondary school students in China, comprising 1,343 in the Mainland and 298 in Hong Kong (Table 6.4). These

Table 6.4 Means of background characteristics and idolizing

Variable	Scoring	Mainland	Hong Kong	All
	N	1343	298	1641
Fan club member	0, 100	5.8	8.2	6.2
Secondary school grade	1–6	3.2	2.5	3.0
Age	years	15.4	14.1	15.1
Female	0, 100	49.5	62.9	51.9
Paternal grade	1–6	4.0	2.7	3.8
Maternal grade	1–6	3.8	2.6	3.6
Idolizing	0–100	46.5	40.0	45.3
Idol modeling	0–100	60.5	45.2	57.7
Idol romanticizing	0–100	22.1	24.7	22.6
Idol idealizing	0–100	42.4	37.9	41.6
Idol commodifying	0–100	37.8	37.4	37.7
Idol befriending	0–100	63.0	50.3	60.7
Idol faming	0–100	41.2	30.9	39.3
Idol crediting	0–100	51.5	40.1	49.4
Idol glamourizing	0–100	52.8	42.6	50.9
Idol beautifying	0–100	43.6	45.3	43.9
Idol popularizing	0–100	9.4	18.0	10.9
Idol personalizing	0–100	87.7	69.2	84.4
Idol glorifying	0–100	47.2	39.7	45.9
Idol prizing	0–100	41.3	37.5	40.6
Idol acceptance	0–100	84.8	77.2	83.5
Model acceptance	0–100	78.7	69.6	77.2

Note
The parental grade had 1 for no school, 2 for primary school, 3 for secondary school, 4 for matriculation, 5 for college, and 6 for graduate school.

..o were an average of 15.1 years old and 3.0 in the secondary school grade. ..mong them, 51.9% were female and 6.2% identified themselves as members of fan clubs. The students' parents, on average, attained a secondary school level (*m* = 3.8–4.0). These students responded to a survey questionnaire to rate items of idolatry and features of their idols (i.e., three idols nominated by each student), self-efficacy, attachment style, and intimacy on some rating scales (see Tables 6.4–6.6). For ease of interpretation and comparison, all the scales generated scores on a 0–100 scale, with 0 for the lowest point, 50 for the midpoint, and 100 for the highest point.

Among idols nominated by the students, 50.3% were star idols, 43.9% were entertainment idols, 28.8% were female idols, 71.2% were male idols, 25.8% were luminary idols, and 23.9% were historical idols (Table 6.5). The less common

Table 6.5 Means of idol features

Variable	Scoring	Mainland	Hong Kong	All
	N	1,343	298	1,641
Western idol	0, 100	17.5	3.6	13.9
Japanese idol	0, 100	1.9	5.6	2.9
Female idol	0, 100	24.5	44.0	28.8
Entertainment idol	0, 100	38.3	68.8	43.9
Athletic idol	0, 100	7.2	0.4	6.0
Academic idol	0, 100	5.9	0.1	4.8
Ideological idol	0, 100	0.4	0.0	0.4
Literary idol	0, 100	4.2	1.0	3.7
Political idol	0, 100	15.1	1.3	12.6
Military idol	0, 100	2.3	0.0	1.8
Business idol	0, 100	4.1	1.6	3.6
Historical idol	0, 100	28.6	3.2	23.9
Fictional idol	0, 100	0.7	1.7	0.9
Familial idol	0, 100	5.9	1.0	5.0
Parent idol	0, 100	4.2	0.7	3.5
Teacher idol	0, 100	1.1	1.0	1.1
Peer idol	0, 100	2.3	0.8	2.0
Heroic idol	0, 100	2.0	0.3	1.7
Altruistic idol	0, 100	0.2	3.0	0.9
Idealistic idol	0, 100	0.1	2.7	0.8
Scientist idol	0, 100	5.7	0.0	4.6
Musical idol	0, 100	0.9	0.1	0.8
Mathematics idol	0, 100	0.0	0.1	0.0
Professional idol	0, 100	0.1	0.0	0.1
Artistic idol	0, 100	1.2	0.1	1.0
Navigating idol	0, 100	0.1	0.0	0.1
Criminal idol	0, 100	0.5	1.1	0.6
Star idol	0, 100	46.0	69.8	50.3
Luminary idol	0, 100	30.9	2.6	25.8
Noncelebrity idol	0, 100	12.3	4.1	10.8

ones were Western idols (13.9%), political idols (12.6%), and at...
(6.0%). Notably, whereas 10.8% were noncelebrity idols, 89.2% were celeb.
idols. Therefore, idols and celebrities were almost equivalent.

Idolizing comprised the following 11 components with 25 items (see Table 6.4). Among the components, idol personalizing was the highest, at a very high level ($m = 84.4$, see Table 6.4), whereas idol popularizing was the lowest, at a very low level ($m = 10.9$). There were relatively high levels of idol befriending ($m = 60.7$), idol modeling ($m = 57.7$), and idol glamourizing ($m = 50.9$). In addition to the 11 first-order components of idolizing, the two second-order components, idol glorifying and idol prizing, were at a modest level ($m = 45.9$ and 40.6). Furthermore, acceptance of the idol as an idol and model were very high ($m = 83.5$ and 77.2).

Modeling

1   Wishing to be able to be someone like my idol
10 Regarding my idol as an example of my personal striving
11 Feeling an invisible force inspiring me, whenever thinking of my idol

Romanticizing

2   Wishing to be able to be my idol's lover
12 Regarding my idol as my dreamed lover
21 Imagining my idol loving me too

Idealizing

3   Thinking that my idol is the most perfect person in the world
14 Thinking that my idol is the most capable person in the world
13 Thinking that my idol is irreplaceable

Commodifying

4   Spending money on things related to my idol
15 Never caring about spending money on my idol
26 Liking to buy things related to my idol

Befriending

5   Wishing to be able to be my idol's friend
16 Imagining to be able to meet and talk freely with my idol
22 Feeling my idol being as kind as my sibling

Faming

24 Choosing idols according to their fame
23 Wishing to be able to be as impressive as my idol

Crediting

6 Thinking that an idol should be successful
17 Choosing idols according to their success in career

Glamourizing

7 Wishing to be able to be as glamorous as my idol
18 Choosing idols according to their glamour

Beautifying

9 Thinking that a male idol should be tall and handsome
20 Thinking that a female idol should be pretty

Popularizing

8 Choosing my idol according to my friends' liking
19 Choosing my idol according to the liking of my parents and/or teachers

Personalizing

25 Choosing idols according to my personal decision

In addition, factor analysis revealed that idol glorifying and prizing subsume eight of the above idolizing components. Accordingly, idol glorifying comprised idol glamourizing, beautifying, faming, and crediting (see Table 6.3). Idol prizing comprised idol commodifying, idealizing, befriending, and romanticizing. Meanwhile, idol modeling, popularizing, and personalizing remained separate components.

Generalized perceived self-efficacy combined the following ten items (Schwarzer et al. 1999). It was at a modest level ($m = 56.4$, see Table 6.6).

1 I can always manage to solve difficult problems if I try hard enough.
2 If someone opposes me, I can find means and ways to get what I want.
3 It is easy for me to stick to my aims and accomplish my goals.

Table 6.6 Means of self-efficacy, attachment style, and intimacy

Variable	Scoring	Mainland	Hong Kong	All
	N	1,343	298	1,641
Self-efficacy	0–100	57.8	49.9	56.4
Secure attachment	0–100	57.5	49.6	56.0
Preoccupied attachment	0–100	47.4	48.6	47.6
Dismissive attachment	0–100	56.1	47.1	54.4
Fearful attachment	0–100	37.6	43.1	38.7
Intimacy	0–100	69.0	59.8	67.4
Frank intimacy	0–100	73.2	65.0	71.8
Sensitive intimacy	0–100	70.3	62.2	68.9
Attaching intimacy	0–100	69.4	55.8	67.1
Exclusive intimacy	0–100	62.9	54.3	61.4
Sharing intimacy	0–100	73.8	62.5	71.9
Imposing intimacy	0–100	60.8	55.9	59.9
Partnering intimacy	0–100	73.2	62.6	71.4
Trustful intimacy	0–100	67.9	59.1	66.4

4 I am confident that I could deal efficiently with unexpected events.
5 Thanks to my resourcefulness, I know how to handle unforeseen situations.
6 I can solve most problems if I invest the necessary effort.
7 I can remain calm when facing difficulties because I can rely on my coping abilities.
8 When I am confronted with a problem, I can usually find several solutions.
9 If I am in trouble, I can usually think of something to do.
10 No matter what comes my way, I am usually able to handle it.

Attachment style, based on the Attachment Style Questionnaire, comprised the following items for the four styles: dismissive, fearful, preoccupied, and secure attachment (Feeney et al. 1994). Secure attachment ($m = 56.0$, see Table 6.6) and dismissive attachment ($m = 54.4$) appeared to be higher than fearful attachment ($m = 38.7$) and preoccupied attachment ($m = 47.6$).

Dismissive attachment

4 I prefer to depend on myself rather than other people.
9 Doing your best is more important than getting along with others.
10 If you've got a job to do, you should do it no matter who gets hurt.
16 I find it hard to trust other people.
19 I find it relatively easy to get close to other people.
34 Other people have their own problems, so I don't bother them with mine.
39 I get frustrated when others are not available when I need them.

Fearful attachment

5   I prefer to keep to myself.
21   I feel comfortable depending on other people.
22   I worry that others won't care about me as much as I care about them.
23   I worry about people getting too close.
27   I wonder why people would want to be involved with me.
30   I wonder how I would cope without someone to love me.
33   I often worry that I do not really fit in with other people.
37   If something is bothering me, others are generally aware and concerned.
40   Other people often disappoint me.

Preoccupied attachment

12   It's important to me to avoid doing things that others won't like.
13   I find it hard to make a decision unless I know what other people think.
15   Sometimes I think I am no good at all.
18   I find that others are reluctant to get as close as I would like.
20   I find it easy to trust others.
26   While I want to get close to others, I feel uneasy about it.
28   It's very important to me to have a close relationship.
31   I feel confident about relating to others.
38   I am confident that other people will like and respect me.

Secure attachment

1   Overall, I am a worthwhile person.
3   I feel confident that other people will be there for me when I need them.
6   To ask for help is to admit that you're a failure.
17   I find it difficult to depend on others.
35   When I talk over my problems with others, I generally feel ashamed or foolish.
36   I am too busy with other activities to put much time into relationships.

Intimacy with the closest friend comprised the following 32 items in eight components: frank, sensitive, attaching, sharing, exclusive, imposing, partnering, and trustful intimacy (Sharabany 1994). Overall, intimacy was at a moderately high level ($m = 67.4$, see Table 6.6). Among its components, sharing intimacy ($m = 71.9$), frank intimacy ($m = 71.8$), and partnering intimacy ($m = 71.4$) were the highest. In contrast, imposing intimacy was the lowest ($m = 59.9$).

Frank intimacy: Frankness and spontaneity

1 I feel free to talk with him about almost everything.
2 If he does something which I do not like, I can always talk with him about it.
3 I talk with him about my hopes and plans for the future.
4 I tell him when I have done something that other people would not approve of.

Sensitive intimacy: Sensitivity and knowing

5 I know how he feels about things without his telling me.
6 I know which kinds of books, games, and activities he likes.
7 I know how he feels about the girl he likes.
8 I can tell when he is worried about something.

Attaching intimacy: Attachment

9 I feel close to him.
10 I like him.
11 When he is not around I miss him.
12 When he is not around I keep wondering where he is and what he is doing.

Exclusive intimacy: Exclusiveness

13 The most exciting things happen when I am with him and nobody else is around.
14 I do things with him that are quite different from what other kids do.
15 It bothers me to have other kids come around and join in when the two of us are doing something together.
16 I stay with him when he wants to do something that other children do not want to do.

Sharing intimacy: Giving and sharing

17 When something nice happens to me I share the experience with him.
18 Whenever he wants to tell me about a problem I stop what I am doing and listen for as long as he wants.
19 I offer him the use of my things (like clothes, toys, food, or books).
20 If he wants something I let him have it even if I want it too.

Imposing intimacy: Imposition

21 I can be sure he'll help me whenever I ask for it.
22 I can plan how we'll spend our time without having to check with him.

23 If I want him to do something for me all I have to do is ask.
24 I can use his things without asking permission.

Partnering intimacy: Common activities

25 Whenever you see me you can be pretty sure that he is also around.
26 I like to do things with him.
27 I work with him on some of his hobbies.
28 I work with him on some of his school work.

Trusting intimacy: Trust and loyalty

29 I know that whatever I tell him is kept secret between us.
30 I will not go along with others to do anything against him.
31 I speak up to defend him when other kids say bad things about him.
32 I tell people nice things about him.

Internal consistency reliability in all composites was satisfactory. Among idolizing composites, the reliability was highest in overall idolizing ($\alpha = .815$, Table 6.7) and lowest in idol faming ($\alpha = .444$). Idol acceptance and model acceptance of accepting the three nominated idols as idols and models respectively also exhibited good reliability ($\alpha = .777$ and .698). Notably, idol personalizing had no internal consistency reliability because it was composed of one item only. Among composites of self-efficacy, attachment style, and intimacy with the closest friend, the reliability was highest in overall intimacy ($\alpha = .941$, Table 6.8) and lowest in secure attachment ($\alpha = .476$).

Table 6.7 Reliability of idolizing

Composite	Number of items	Raw	Standard
Idol modeling	3	.743	.741
Idol romanticizing	3	.783	.791
Idol idealizing	3	.775	.776
Idol commodifying	3	.789	.788
Idol befriending	3	.726	.729
Idol faming	2	.444	.451
Idol crediting	2	.554	.554
Idol glamourizing	2	.572	.572
Idol beautifying	2	.655	.657
Idol popularizing	2	.553	.558
Idol personalizing	1	-	-
Idolizing	11	.815	.810
Idol glorifying	4	.733	.735
Idol prizing	4	.742	.742
Idol acceptance	3	.777	.778
Model acceptance	3	.698	.699

Table 6.8 Reliability of self-efficacy, attachment style, and intimacy

Composite	Number of items	Raw	Standard
Self-efficacy	10	.857	.857
Intimacy	32	.941	.943
Frank intimacy	4	.717	.718
Sensitive intimacy	4	.722	.723
Attaching intimacy	4	.770	.771
Exclusive intimacy	4	.576	.585
Sharing intimacy	4	.745	.749
Imposing intimacy	4	.629	.634
Partnering intimacy	4	.731	.734
Trustful intimacy	4	.664	.672
Secure attachment	6	.476	.485
Preoccupied attachment	10	.788	.787
Dismissive attachment	7	.556	.556
Fearful attachment	9	.716	.716

Relationships between idolizing, self-efficacy, attachment style, intimacy, and idol features

Relationships between idolizing, self-efficacy, attachment style, intimacy, and idol features derive from partial correlations controlling for all background characteristics and the response set of acquiescence. Acquiescence was the average of all rating items to signify the tendency toward a high rating regardless of item content. The correlations applied to all students and their subgroups, including male and female students, early adolescents (aged below 15 years) and older adolescents (aged 15 years or above), and Mainland and Hong Kong Chinese.

Idolizing generally had negative relationships with self-efficacy belief, secure attachment, and intimacy with the closest friend. The strongest relationship was between idolizing and dismissive attachment (partial $r = -.196$, Table 6.9) and sharing intimacy (partial $r = -.193$). Moreover, idolizing maintained significant negative relationships with intimacy and self-efficacy (partial $r = -.183$ and $-.066$). The relationships supported the compensation thesis as opposed to the spillover thesis about idolizing as a compensation for deficiency in self-efficacy, attachment, and intimacy. That is, when idolizing was lower, self-efficacy, attachment, and intimacy were higher. In other words, idolizing and relationships with self and others were mutually exclusive.

Relationships between idolizing and self-efficacy were stronger in an inverse way in the female, older, or Hong Kong student than in the male, younger, or Mainland student. That is, compensation between idolizing and self-efficacy was greater in the female, older, or Hong Kong student. The relationship was most negative in the Hong Kong student (partial $r = -.301$, see Table 6.9). In contrast, idolizing had virtually no relationship with self-efficacy in the early adolescent, male student, and Mainland Chinese (partial $r = -.003, .010,$ and $-.022$).

Table 6.9 Partial correlations between idolizing and self-efficacy, attachment style, and intimacy

Correlate	All	Male	Female	Early	Older	Main-land	Hong Kong
Self-efficacy	−.066**	.010	−.217**	−.003	−.169**	−.022	−.301**
Secure attachment	−.033	.100	−.148**	.169**	−.178**	−.032	−.124
Preoccupied attachment	−.053	.055	−.202**	.043	−.180**	−.034	−.237**
Dismissive attachment	−.196**	−.048	−.377**	−.032	−.370**	−.201**	−.341**
Fearful attachment	−.189**	−.051	−.394**	−.123*	−.305**	−.206**	−.277**
Intimacy	−.122**	−.038	−.466**	.030	−.526**	.008	−.945**
Frank intimacy	−.183**	−.146**	−.339**	−.064	−.372**	−.096˙	−.789**
Sensitive intimacy	−.131**	−.069	−.359**	.016	−.422**	−.056	−.741**
Attaching intimacy	−.101**	−.001	−.372**	.029	−.383**	.008	−.786**
Exclusive intimacy	−.008	.073	−.232**	.090	−.243**	.076	−.678**
Sharing intimacy	−.193**	−.160**	−.402**	−.067	−.476**	−.096˙	−.866**
Imposing intimacy	.021	.033	−.162**	.099	−.192**	.099˙	−.657**
Partnering intimacy	−.104**	−.047	−.366**	−.006	−.368**	.031	−.845**
Trusting intimacy	−.040	.059	−.264**	.080	−.273**	.060	−.704**

Notes
*$p < .05$
**$p < .01$

Relationships between idolizing and secure attachment were stronger in an inverse way in the female, older, or Hong Kong student than in the male, younger, or Mainland student. Notably, idolizing exhibited the strongest negative relationship with secure attachment in the older adolescent (partial $r = -.178$, see Table 6.9).

However, idolizing also showed significant negative correlations with insecure attachment in terms of dismissive attachment and fearful attachment (partial $r = -.196$ and $-.189$, see Table 6.9). The negative correlations were stronger in the female student, older adolescent, and Hong Kong Chinese than in others. These negative correlations suggest that insecure attachment reduces idolizing or vice versa. Such a relationship espouses the spillover thesis about spillover between the idol and people in general.

Relationships between idolizing and intimacy with the closest friend were stronger in an inverse way in the female, older, or Hong Kong student than in the male, younger, or Mainland student. Notably, the relationship was very strong in Hong Kong (partial $r = -.945$, see Table 6.9). Clearly, idolizing appears to be a compensation for intimacy with the closest friend or vice versa. In contrast, relationships between idolizing and intimacy with the closest friend were minimal in the male student, early adolescent, and Mainland Chinese (partial $r = -.038$, .030, and .008). That is, compensation between idolizing and intimacy did not happen in the male student, early adolescent, and Mainland Chinese.

Idolizing showed very weak positive relationships with idol acceptance and model acceptance (partial $r = .093$ and .068, see Table 6.10). The relationships were stronger in the male student, early adolescent, and Mainland Chinese (partial $r = .143, .132,$ and $.116; .012, .092,$ and $.067$). Obviously, acceptance as the idol or model is different from idolizing.

Idolizing had significant relationships with some idol features. Accordingly, idolizing was higher in the entertainment idol and star idol than in the others (partial $r = .141$ and $.150$, see Table 6.10). In contrast, idolizing was lower in the historical idol, parent as an idol, luminary idol, and idol who was not a celebrity (partial $r = -.068, -.054, -.062,$ and $-.053$). The entertainment idol and star

Table 6.10 Partial correlations between idolizing and idol features

Correlate	All	Male	Female	Early	Older	Mainland	Hong Kong
Idol acceptance	.093**	.143**	.022	.132**	.042	.116**	.022
Model acceptance	.068**	.102**	.031	.092*	.056	.067*	.052
Western idol	−.017	−.044	−.012	−.009	−.040	−.034	.017
Japanese idol	.022	.039	.001	.003	.042	.045	−.040
Female idol	.047	.111*	−.006	.049	.017	.040	.029
Entertainment idol	.141**	.158**	.100**	.153**	.107**	.131**	.153*
Athletic idol	.026	.022	.025	.031	.019	.025	.020
Academic idol	−.019	−.010	−.039	−.024	−.008	−.025	.056
Ideological idol	−.029	−.054	−.002	.020	−.066	−.037	.
Literary idol	−.019	.021	−.044	−.023	−.004	−.027	.007
Political idol	−.019	.000	−.040	−.004	−.045	−.027	.015
Military idol	−.029	−.030	−.039	−.024	−.041	−.035	.
Business idol	.006	.023	−.026	.014	.008	.003	.019
Historical idol	−.068**	−.065	−.069	−.065	−.068*	−.081**	−.020
Fictional idol	.001	−.022	.027	.007	−.007	.006	−.039
Familial idol	−.040	−.049	−.020	−.052	−.009	−.035	−.076
Parent idol	−.054*	−.055	−.038	−.053	−.036	−.050	−.082
Teacher idol	−.013	−.015	−.011	−.003	−.037	−.002	−.054
Peer idol	−.015	−.043	.016	−.018	.007	−.014	−.039
Heroic idol	−.042	−.057	−.025	−.056	−.006	−.047	.022
Altruistic idol	.006	−.043	.056	.034	.010	.022	.014
Idealistic idol	−.002	−.043	.040	.034	−.020	.015	−.006
Scientist idol	−.023	−.015	−.039	−.027	−.014	−.028	.
Musical idol	−.022	−.027	−.020	.009	−.062	−.026	.005
Mathematics idol	.004	.004	.	.	.016	−.013	.056
Professional idol	.011	.022	.008	.006	.025	.012	.
Artistic idol	−.022	−.029	−.016	.002	−.048	−.027	.005
Navigating idol	.002	.006	−.003	.008	−.001	.001	.
Criminal idol	.006	.017	−.018	−.022	.032	.006	.025
Star idol	.150**	.164**	.108**	.163**	.115**	.140**	.166**
Luminary idol	−.062*	−.043	−.083*	−.048	−.077*	−.078**	.018
Noncelebrity idol	−.053*	−.081*	−.009	−.055	−.028	−.051	−.085

Notes
*$p < .05$
**$p < .01$

idol earned more idolizing by the male student, early adolescent, and Hong Kong Chinese than by others. Also, the historical idol received less idolizing from Mainland Chinese than Hong Kong Chinese. The luminary idol gained less idolizing from the female student, older adolescent, and Mainland Chinese than from the others. Moreover, the noncelebrity idol attained less idolizing from the boy than from the girl.

Idol glorifying displayed inverse relationships with self-efficacy, attachment styles, and intimacy with the closest friend. These relationships largely support the compensation thesis that idol glorifying is a compensation for deficiency in self, attachment, and intimacy. Notably, the strongest negative relationship was between idol glorifying and sharing intimacy (partial $r = -.243$). In addition, idol glorifying had a significant positive correlation with preoccupied attachment, which means an inadequate self together with insecure attachment (partial $r = .099$). This relationship accords with the compensation thesis, such that inadequate attachment is compatible with idolizing in terms of idol glorifying. The negative relationship or compensation was generally stronger in the female student, older adolescent, and Hong Kong Chinese than in the others. Nevertheless, the linkage between idol glorifying and preoccupied attachment was stronger in the male student, early adolescent, and Mainland Chinese than in the others (partial $r = .161, .134,$ and $.118$).

Idol glorifying had significant correlations with some idol features. Accordingly, positive correlations involved the female idol, entertainment idol, and star idol (partial $r = .077, .163,$ and $.170$). These correlations were stronger in the early adolescent than in the others. Meanwhile, negative correlations involved model acceptance, the historical idol, familial idol, parent idol, heroic idol, luminary idol, and noncelebrity idol (partial $r = -.073, -.089, -.054, -.064, -.063, -.083,$ and $-.088$). The correlation with model acceptance was stronger in the female student, older adolescent, and Mainland Chinese than in the others. In contrast, the correlation with the heroic idol was stronger in the male student, early adolescent, and Mainland Chinese than in the others. The correlation with the luminary idol was stronger in the female student and Mainland Chinese than in the others. In addition, the correlation with the noncelebrity idol was stronger in the male student and early adolescent than in the others. In all, idol glorifying had the strongest positive correlation with the star idol (partial $r = .170$). This means that the star idol receives the most glorification from the student. Furthermore, the correlation was the highest in the early adolescent (partial $r = .199$). This means that the early adolescent glorifies the star idol the most.

Idol prizing manifested significant correlations with self-efficacy, attachment styles, and intimacy with the closest friend. Notably, idol prizing had the strongest negative correlation with dismissive attachment (partial $r = -.202$). This correlation was stronger in the female student, older adolescent, and Hong Kong Chinese than in the others (partial $r = -.367, -.346,$ and $-.368$). Meanwhile, idol prizing had significant negative correlations with self-efficacy, frank intimacy, and sharing intimacy (partial $r = -.074, -.089,$ and $-.105$). The correlations were also stronger in the female student, early adolescent, and Hong Kong Chinese than in the others. Moreover, idol prizing indicated a significant negative correlation with secure attachment in the female student and older adolescent (partial $r = -.161$ and $-.181$). Moreover, idol prizing had a significant negative correlation with overall intimacy in the female student, older adolescent, and Hong Kong Chinese (partial $r = -.336$, $-.320$, and $-.808$). These correlations support the compensation thesis about the contrast between idol prizing and deficiency in self, attachment, and intimacy. Nevertheless, idol prizing maintained a significant positive correlation in the male student and early adolescent (partial $r = .111$ and $.179$). Moreover, the correlation with intimacy was significantly positive in the Mainland student (partial $r = .084$). These correlations endorse the spillover thesis.

Idol prizing showed significant correlations with some idol features. Its correlations were with idol acceptance, model acceptance, the entertainment idol, and the star idol. Thus, idol prizing was compatible with idol and model acceptance (partial $r = .155$ and $.102$). The correlation with idol acceptance was stronger in the male student, early adolescent, and Mainland Chinese than in the others (partial $r = .181$, $.172$, and $.174$). Meanwhile, the correlation with model acceptance was stronger in the male student, older adolescent, and Hong Kong Chinese (partial $r = .130$, $.119$, and $.128$). Idol prizing was most likely for the entertainment idol and star idol. It happened more often in the male student than in the others (partial $r = .157$). In contrast, idol prizing was lower for the historical idol and luminary idol (partial $r = -.089$ and $-.087$). This lower likelihood was particularly evident in the older adolescent and Mainland Chinese.

Idol modeling showed negative correlations with intimacy with the closest friend. These correlations support the compensation thesis that idolizing and intimacy with friends are compensatory to each other. Particularly, there were significant negative correlations between idol modeling and exclusive intimacy and imposing intimacy (partial $r = -.114$ and $-.079$). Negative correlations were stronger in the female student, older adolescent, and Hong Kong Chinese than in the others.

In contrast, idol modeling displayed positive correlations with self-efficacy and secure attachment and negative correlations with fearful attachment and preoccupied attachment (partial $r = .052$, $.055$, $-.208$, and $-.159$). These correlations were in line with the spillover thesis as opposed to the compensation thesis. Thus, self-efficacy and secure attachment extended to idol modeling or vice versa. This spillover effect thus differentiated idol modeling from other components of idolizing. Specifically, whereas spillover between idol modeling and self-efficacy were significant in the male student and Mainland Chinese (partial $r = .095$ and $.102$), compensation between idol modeling and self-efficacy were significant in the Hong Kong Chinese (partial $r = -.209$). Moreover, significant spillover between idol modeling and secure attachment appeared in the early adolescent only (partial $r = .154$). Inverse relationships between idol modeling and preoccupied and fearful attachment were stronger in the female student and older adolescent.

Idol modeling manifested significant correlations with some idol features. The correlations with idol acceptance and model acceptance were positive, indicating compatibility between idol modeling and acceptance (partial $r = .132$ and $.262$).

This compatibility was stronger in the male student, early adolescent, and Mainland Chinese than in their counterparts. Idol modeling also maintained positive correlations with the Western idol, academic idol, political idol, historical idol, altruistic idol, scientist idol, and luminary idol. That is, these idols received more idol modeling from the student. Among them, the luminary idol received the highest idol modeling (partial r = .150). Conversely, idol modeling was lower in the female idol, entertainment idol, and star idol than in others (partial r = −.087, −.172, and −.161).

Idol romanticizing displayed negative correlations with self-efficacy, secure attachment, and intimacy with the closest friend (partial r = −.066, −.058, and −.105). These correlations support the compensation thesis, which posits compensation or displacement between idolizing and other relationships. Notably, compensation between idol romanticizing and self-efficacy was greater in the female student, older adolescent, and Hong Kong Chinese than in the others (partial r = −.191, −.112, and −.175). Likewise, compensation between idol romanticizing and intimacy was significant in the female student, older adolescent, and Hong Kong Chinese (partial r = −.311, −.321, and −.544). In addition, compensation between idol romanticizing and secure attachment was significant in the female student and older adolescent (partial r = −.125 and −.129). Nevertheless, idol romanticizing showed a significant negative correlation with dismissive attachment (partial r = −.155). This indicates a spillover between dismissive attachment and dismissal from idol romanticizing. Such spillover was stronger in the female student, older adolescent, and Hong Kong Chinese than in the others (partial r = −.249, −.229, and −.246).

Idol romanticizing did not show significant correlations with idol and model acceptance (partial r = .011 and −.012). Hence, idol romanticizing was independent of model acceptance.

Idol romanticizing had significant correlations with some idol features. Positive correlations indicate that idol romanticizing was higher for the female idol, entertainment idol, and star idol than for the others (partial r = .064, .162, and .152). The higher idol romanticizing for the female idol was particularly evident in the male student and Mainland Chinese (partial r = .218 and .088). In addition, the entertainment idol and star idol received greater romanticizing from the male student, older adolescent, and Mainland Chinese than from the other. In contrast, negative correlations show that the political idol, military idol, historical idol, and luminary idol received less romanticizing than did the others (partial r = −.060, −.055, −.099, and −.104).

Idol idealizing exhibited nonsignificant negative correlations with self-efficacy, secure attachment, and intimacy with the closest friend (partial r = −.047, −.040, and −.002). However, the negative correlations were significant in the female student and older adolescent. The Hong Kong Chinese also had significant negative correlations between idol idealizing and self-efficacy and intimacy with the closest friend (partial r = −.190 and −.533). These negative correlations support the compensation thesis about displacement between idol idealizing and relationships with others.

Idol idealizing also showed significant negative correlation with insecure attachment in terms of preoccupied, dismissive, and fearful attachment (partial $r = .064, .162,$ and $.152$). These correlations suggest spillover between attachment security and idol idealizing. The spillover was greater in the female student, older adolescent, and Hong Kong Chinese than in the others.

Idol idealizing had significant positive correlations with idol and model acceptance (partial $r = .184$ and $.155$). Hence, idol idealizing was compatible with acceptance. Idol idealizing, however, did not maintain a significant correlation with any idol features generally. Only the younger adolescent and Hong Kong Chinese showed significant positive correlations between idol idealizing and the altruistic idol and idealistic idol (partial $r = .119$ and $.119$). That is, idealistic and altruistic idols received more idealizing in the younger adolescent and Hong Kong Chinese.

Idol commodifying had negative correlations with self-efficacy and secure attachment (partial $r = -.042$ and $-.047$). The correlations were significant in the female student and older adolescent. Moreover, the female student and Hong Kong Chinese held a significant negative correlation between idol commodifying and intimacy with the closest friend (partial $r = -.139$ and $-.590$). These negative correlations endorse the compensation thesis about compensation between idolizing and other relationships.

Idol commodifying also had significant negative correlations with insecure attachment in terms of preoccupied, dismissive, and fearful attachment (partial $r -.113, -.184,$ and $-.141$). These correlations were stronger in the female student and older adolescent than in the others. Idol commodifying also manifested a significant positive correlation with imposing intimacy (partial $r = .157$). This correlation was stronger in the male student, early adolescent, and Mainland Chinese (partial $r = .136, .186,$ and $.209$). All these correlations support the spillover thesis between idolizing and other relationships.

Idol commodifying showed significant positive correlations with idol and model acceptance (partial $r = .130$ and $.051$). Commodifying was thus compatible with acceptance. Idol commodifying had significant correlations with some idol features. The positive correlations indicate that the entertainment idol and star idol received more idol commodifying than did others (partial $r = .170$ and $.182$). Meanwhile, the negative correlations showed that the political idol, historical idol, familial idol, parent idol, luminary idol, and noncelebrity idol received less idol commodifying than did others (partial $r = -.058, -.094, -.064, -.056, -.089,$ and $-.081$). Obviously, commodifying did not apply to these idols.

Idol befriending maintained a significant negative but weak correlation with self-efficacy (partial $r = -.051$). The negative correlation was stronger in the female student, older adolescent, and Hong Kong Chinese (partial $r = -.134, -.087,$ and $-.226$). These students also manifested a significant negative correlation between idol befriending and self-efficacy (partial $r = -.169, -.231,$ and $-.658$). These negative correlations support the compensation thesis about the trade-off between idolizing and other relationships.

Idol befriending also showed significant negative correlations with dismissive attachment and fearful attachment (partial $r = -.149$ and $-.194$). The correlations were stronger in the female student, older adolescent, and Hong Kong Chinese. Furthermore, the early adolescent exhibited a positive significant correlation between idol befriending and secure attachment (partial $r = .203$). The Mainland student also displayed significant positive correlations between idol befriending and intimacy, particularly attaching intimacy, partnering intimacy, and trusting intimacy (partial $r = .085, .095, .115$, and $.091$). All these correlations support the spillover thesis about generalization across relations.

Idol befriending displayed significant positive correlations with idol and model acceptance (partial $r = .093$ and $.095$). These correlations were stronger in the male student than in the female (partial $r = .152$ and $.134$). Hence, befriending is compatible with acceptance.

Idol befriending had significant correlations with some idol features. On the one hand, the positive correlations indicated that the entertainment idol, teacher idol, and star idol received more idol befriending than did others (partial $r = .090, .053$, and $.091$). Particularly, the entertainment idol and star idol received more idol befriending from the male student and Hong Kong Chinese than from the others. On the other hand, the negative correlations revealed that the historical idol and luminary idol received less idol befriending than did others (partial $r = -.073$ and $-.063$).

Idol faming displayed negative correlations with self-efficacy, secure attachment, and intimacy with the closest friend (partial $r = -.044, -.057$, and $-.125$). The correlations were stronger in the female student, older adolescent, and Hong Kong Chinese than in the others. Conversely, idol faming manifested a positive correlation with insecure attachment in terms of preoccupied attachment (partial $r = .105$). This correlation was stronger in the male student, older adolescent, and Mainland Chinese than in the others (partial $r = .171, .111$, and $.122$). All these correlations sustain the compensation thesis about the trade-off between idolizing and other relationships. Moreover, the female student, older adolescent, and Hong Kong Chinese evinced greater compensation than did others.

Idol faming also had significant negative correlations with dismissive attachment and fearful attachment (partial $r = -.154$ and $-.082$). These correlations endorse the spillover thesis about generalization of relationships. That is, insecure attachment in terms of dismissive and fearful attachment maintained an inverse relationship with idol faming.

Idol faming did not show significant correlation with idol and model acceptance generally (partial $r = -.045$ and $-.049$). Thus, idol faming and acceptance were independent of each other.

Idol faming manifested significant negative correlations with two idol features. According to the correlations, the parent idol and noncelebrity idol received less idol faming (partial $r = -.051$ and $-.057$). Particularly, the heroic idol received less idol faming from the male student, early adolescent, and Mainland Chinese than from others (partial $r = -.078, -.083$, and $-.061$). Meanwhile, the noncelebrity idol received less idol faming from the early adolescent than from the older adolescent (partial $r = -.090$).

Idol crediting manifested negative correlations with self-efficacy, secure attachment, and intimacy with the closest friends. Particularly, the negative correlation with self-efficacy was significant in the Hong Kong Chinese (partial $r = -.214$). In addition, the negative correlation with secure attachment was significant in the older adolescent (partial $r = -.097$). The negative correlation with intimacy was significant in the female student, older adolescent, and Hong Kong Chinese (partial $r = -.291, -.274,$ and $-.603$). All these negative correlations accord with the compensation thesis about compensation between idolizing, self-efficacy, attachment security, and intimacy.

Idol crediting maintained significant correlations with some idol features. The significant negative correlations indicated that the heroic idol and noncelebrity idol received less idol crediting (partial $r = -.056$ and $-.054$). The correlation with the heroic idol was significant in the male student, early adolescent, and Mainland Chinese (partial $r = -.078, -.093,$ and $-.061$). Meanwhile, the negative correlation with the noncelebrity idol was significant in the early adolescent (partial $r = -.090$).

Idol glamourizing presented negative correlations with self-efficacy, secure attachment, and intimacy with the closest friend. The negative correlation with self-efficacy was significant in the female student, older adolescent, and Hong Kong Chinese (partial $r = -.142, -.083,$ and $-.158$). In addition, the negative correlation with secure attachment was significant in the female student (partial $r = -.148$). There were significant negative correlations with overall intimacy in the female student, older adolescent, and Hong Kong Chinese (partial $r = -.256, -.326,$ and $-.610$). All these negative correlations support the compensation thesis, which posits that idolizing is a compensation for inadequate attachment and intimacy or vice versa.

Idol glamourizing, nevertheless, also manifested a significant negative correlation with dismissive attachment (partial $r = -.136$). The correlation was also particularly significant in the female student, older adolescent, and both the Mainland and Hong Kong Chinese (partial $r = -.136, -.270, -.224, -.144,$ and $-.172$). These negative correlations support the spillover thesis, which posits that insecure attachment diminishes idolizing or vice versa.

Idol glamourizing had significant correlations with some idol features. Significant positive correlations showed that the female idol, entertainment idol, and star idol received more idol glamourizing (partial $r = .070, .141,$ and $.150$). Particularly, idol glamourizing of the female idol was significantly higher than for the other idols by the male student and Mainland Chinese (partial $r = .087$ and $.074$). Meanwhile, the significant negative correlations indicate that the academic idol, historical idol, parent as idol, heroic idol, scientist as idol, luminary idol, and noncelebrity idol received less idol glamourizing.

Idol beautifying displayed negative correlations with self-efficacy, secure attachment, and intimacy with the closest friend (partial $r = -.079, -.028,$ and $-.114$). Notably, the negative correlation with self-efficacy was significant in the female student, older adolescent, and both the Mainland and Hong Kong Chinese (partial $r = -.153, -.128, -.066,$ and $-.173$). Meanwhile, the negative correlation with intimacy was greater in the older adolescent and Hong Kong

Chinese (partial $r = -.325$ and $-.536$). Furthermore, idol beautifying displayed a significant positive correlation with preoccupied attachment (partial $r = .078$). Particularly, the positive correlation between idol beautifying and preoccupied attachment was positive in the Mainland Chinese (partial $r = .081$). These correlations endorse the compensation thesis that idolizing and other relationships are compensatory or substitutes to each other. That is, inadequate self-efficacy, attachment, and intimacy were associated with idol beautifying.

Idol beautifying also exhibited a significant negative correlation with dismissive attachment (partial $r = -.181$). This correlation suggests spillover between idol beautifying and nondismissive attachment.

Idol beautifying exhibited a significant negative correlation with acceptance of the idol as a model (partial $r = -.119$). The correlation suggests that idol beautifying and model acceptance are contradictory to each other. This was in favor of the compensatory model about idol beautifying and other relationships.

Idol beautifying had significant correlations with some idol features. On the one hand, significant positive correlations suggest that the female idol, entertainment idol, and star idol received more idol beautifying than did the others (partial $r = .112$, $.230$, and $.228$). On the other hand, significant negative correlations revealed that the Western idol, literary idol, political idol, military idol, historical idol, heroic idol, luminary idol, and noncelebrity idol received less idol beautifying than did others.

Idol popularizing displayed negative correlations with self-efficacy and intimacy with the closest friend (partial $r = -.103$ and $-.051$). The correlation with self-efficacy was stronger in the male student and older adolescent than in the others (partial $r = -.110$ and $-.136$). In addition, the correlation with intimacy was significant in the female student, older adolescent, and Hong Kong Chinese (partial $r = -.135$, $-.104$, and $-.425$). The correlations with frank intimacy and partnering intimacy, particularly, were significant (partial $r = -.105$ and $-.076$). These negative correlations are supportive of the compensatory thesis about compensation between idolizing and other relationships. Nevertheless, idol popularizing did not have a significant correlation with any attachment style.

Idol popularizing indicated a significant negative correlation with idol acceptance (partial $r = -.061$). Particularly, the negative correlation was significant in the female student and older adolescent (partial $r = -.096$ and $-.078$). The negative correlation suggests that idol popularizing and acceptance are contradictory to each other. In addition, idol popularizing did not show a significant correlation with any idol feature.

Idol personalizing displayed significant negative correlations with preoccupied attachment and fearful attachment (partial $r = -.147$ and $-.180$). The correlations were stronger in the female student, older adolescent, and Mainland Chinese. These correlations were consistent with the spillover thesis that inadequate attachment impedes idolizing.

Idol personalizing had significant negative correlations with self-efficacy and intimacy with the closest friend only in the Hong Kong Chinese (partial

$r = -.148$ and $-.234$). These correlations were in line with the compensatory thesis about contradiction between idolizing and other relationships.

Idol personalizing displayed significant positive correlation with model acceptance, the entertainment idol, and the star idol (partial $r = .057$, $.083$, and $.086$). The latter indicates that the entertainment idol and star idol were more associated with idol personalizing than were the others. The association was stronger in the male student, early adolescent, and Hong Kong Chinese than in the others.

Predicting idolatry

Predicting idolatry involved idolizing, acceptance, and various idol features as outcomes and the basic background characteristics of the student's age, school grade, maternal and paternal education, region, and fan club membership as predictors. Linear regression analysis estimated the net effects of the predictors on each of the outcomes.

Concerning idolizing and acceptance, significant background differences were as follows. Significant effects showed that the female student displayed greater idol romanticizing and befriending than did the male student ($\beta = .052$ and $.072$, Table 6.11). However, other significant effects indicated that the female student was lower in idol faming, idol acceptance, and model acceptance than was the male student ($\beta = -.090$, $-.066$, and $-.062$). The older student had higher romanticizing but lower befriending ($\beta = .107$ and $-.088$). The student in a higher school grade displayed lower idol popularizing ($\beta = -.301$). One

Table 6.11 Standardized regression coefficients of idolizing

Outcome	Fan club member	Grade	Age	Female	Dad grade	Mom grade	Hong Kong	R^2
Idolizing	.152***	.000	.019	-.008	.041	.025	-.129***	.050
Idol glorifying	.094***	.005	.025	-.031	.013	.001	-.122***	.029
Idol prizing	.182***	.015	-.003	.035	.055	.026	-.051	.043
Idol modeling	.062*	-.011	-.069	-.056	.012	.067	-.200***	.065
Idol romanticizing	.116***	-.003	.107*	.052*	.069	.029	.090**	.030
Idol idealizing	.095***	.031	-.051	-.035	.000	.048	-.050	.018
Idol commodifying	.211***	.009	.027	.024	.078*	-.014	.016	.049
Idol befriending	.127***	.013	-.088*	.072**	.020	.015	-.195***	.058
Idol faming	.068**	.001	-.062	-.090***	.012	-.014	-.163***	.041
Idol crediting	.055*	-.057	.082	-.023	.045	.022	-.118***	.033
Idol glamourizing	.096***	.043	.048	.024	.042	-.009	-.107***	.034
Idol beautifying	.060*	.021	.000	-.009	-.054	.006	.008	.007
Idol popularizing	.030	-.116**	.061	-.087	.030	.017	.200***	.051
Idol personalizing	.058*	.048	.072	.054	.029	-.007	-.227***	.083
Idol acceptance	.072**	-.044	.055	-.066**	.025	.077*	-.126***	.049
Model acceptance	.034	-.008	.003	-.062*	-.008	.071*	-.144***	.038

Notes
*$p < .05$
**$p < .01$
***$p < .001$

whose father's school grade was higher was higher in idol commodifying ($\beta = .078$). When the mother's school grade was higher, acceptance of the idol as an idol and model was higher ($\beta = .077$ and $.071$). The Hong Kong Chinese showed lower idolizing, most of its components, and idol and model acceptance than did the Mainland Chinese. Meanwhile, the fan club member held greater idolizing, most of its components, and idol acceptance than did the nonmember.

Regarding the prediction of idol features, background characteristics manifested the following significant differences. The female student was more likely than was the male student to have a female idol, entertainment idol, literary idol, and star idol ($\beta = .230, .134, .069$, and $.062$, Table 6.12). Meanwhile, the female

Table 6.12 Standardized regression coefficients of idol features

Outcome	Fan club member	Grade	Age	Female	Dad grade	Mom grade	Hong Kong	R^2
Western idol	−.032	.047	.033	−.218***	.021	.022	−.119**	.081
Japanese idol	.020	.056	−.005	.031	−.022	.005	.095*	.014
Female idol	.042	−.046	−.050	.230***	−.053	−.044	.099**	.094
Entertainment idol	.085**	−.048	−.036	.134***	−.037	−.051	.172***	.088
Athletic idol	−.004	.075	.014	−.151***	−.026	.019	−.080**	.040
Academic idol	−.034	−.009	−.090	−.030	.014	−.044	−.136***	.021
Ideological idol	−.017	−.003	.021	−.036	.030	−.024	−.017	.003
Literary idol	−.004	.024	−.004	.069**	−.024	.045	−.064*	.011
Political idol	−.032	.025	.063	−.019	.030	−.016	−.129***	.033
Military idol	−.018	−.001	.054	−.084**	.017	.018	−.028	.014
Business idol	−.015	.064	−.024	−.094***	.039	−.016	−.030	.013
Historical idol	−.064*	−.030	.016	−.067**	.028	−.011	−.216***	.062
Fictional idol	.010	.014	−.012	−.016	−.028	.039	.041	.003
Familial idol	.010	−.030	.014	.033	.013	.075*	−.063*	.016
Parent idol	−.007	−.009	−.010	.016	.011	.071*	−.052	.012
Teacher idol	−.014	−.015	−.010	.005	.036	.021	.010	.004
Peer idol	−.015	−.041	−.069	.018	−.009	−.018	−.079**	.012
Heroic idol	−.009	−.036	−.012	−.006	−.019	.036	−.052	.005
Altruistic idol	−.027	.065	−.033	−.043	.025	−.012	.141**	.021
Idealistic idol	−.027	.051	−.039	−.061	.016	−.008	.141**	.023
Scientist idol	−.036	−.014	−.087	−.029	.006	−.041	−.139***	.022
Musical idol	.000	.059	−.076	.024	−.013	.018	−.049	.004
Mathematics idol	−.008	−.033	.040	−.023	.024	−.018	.027	.002
Professional idol	−.008	−.045	.040	.002	.011	−.009	−.009	.001
Artistic idol	−.004	.046	−.054	.020	−.008	.013	−.049	.003
Navigating idol	−.007	.054	−.051	−.017	−.021	.025	−.016	.002
Criminal idol	−.011	−.029	.037	−.050	−.006	.029	.051	.005
Star idol	.084**	−.013	−.029	.062*	−.052	−.041	.133***	.050
Luminary idol	−.055*	.015	.012	−.020	.023	−.021	−.239***	.067
Noncelebrity idol	−.018	−.065	.018	.036	.006	.064	−.088**	.019
Fan club member	−	−.064	−.003	−.072**	.044	−.016	.042	.013

Notes
*$p < .05$
**$p < .01$
***$p < .001$

student was less likely than was the male student to hold a Western idol, athletic idol, military idol, business idol, or historical idol and to be a member of a fan club (β = −.218, −.151, −.084, −.094, −.067, and −.072). When the mother's education was higher, the student was more likely to have a familial idol and parent idol (β = .075 and .071). The Hong Kong Chinese was more likely than was the Mainland Chinese to adore a Japanese idol, female idol, entertainment idol, altruistic idol, idealistic idol, or star idol (β = .095, .099, .172, .141, .141, and .133). Conversely, the Hong Kong Chinese was less likely than was the Mainland Chinese to favor a Western idol, academic idol, political idol, historical idol, familial idol, peer idol, scientist idol, luminary idol, or noncelebrity idol. In addition, the fan club member was more likely than was the nonmember to cherish an entertainment idol or star idol (β = .085 and .084). In addition, the fan club member was less likely than was the nonmember to nominate a historical idol or luminary idol (β = −.064 and −.084).

As regards self-efficacy, attachment style, and intimacy with the closest friend, background characteristics indicated the following significant differences. The female student exhibited higher preoccupied attachment, intimacy, and most of its components than did the male student (β = .083 and .144, Table 6.13). In addition, the female student was lower than was the male student in self-efficacy (β = −.177). The older student had higher dismissive attachment and imposing intimacy (β = .185 and .179). The student of a higher school grade was higher

Table 6.13 Standardized regression coefficients of self-efficacy, attachment style, and intimacy

Outcome	Fan club member	Grade	Age	Female	Dad grade	Mom grade	Hong Kong	R^2
Self-efficacy	.036	−.103*	.022	−.177***	.135***	.077*	−.080**	.108
Secure attachment	.074*	−.005	.073	−.019	.086	.026	−.128**	.051
Preoccupied attachment	−.073*	.090	−.062	.083*	−.144**	.086	−.006	.020
Dismissive attachment	−.006	−.049	.185**	.025	.027	−.041	−.166***	.064
Fearful attachment	−.038	−.087	.050	−.052	−.079	−.018	.095*	.028
Intimacy	.007	.023	.000	.144***	.121*	.041	−.176***	.088
Frank intimacy	.012	.119	−.094	.095**	.131**	−.028	−.153***	.055
Sensitive intimacy	−.022	.123*	−.079	.143***	.134**	−.010	−.131**	.066
Attaching intimacy	−.018	.006	−.051	.154***	.091	.039	−.227***	.098
Exclusive intimacy	.048	−.025	.048	.109**	.123*	.063	−.114**	.069
Sharing intimacy	−.032	.000	.030	.136***	.098*	.021	−.186***	.080
Imposing intimacy	.030	−.097	.179**	.060	.084	.030	−.029	.032
Partnering intimacy	.019	.001	−.064	.068	.047	.088	−.196***	.070
Trustful intimacy	.036	.009	.045	.160***	.058	.088	−.125**	.071

Notes
*$p < .05$
**$p < .01$
***$p < .001$

in sensitive intimacy and lower in self-efficacy (β = .123 and −.103). The student with higher paternal education was higher in self-efficacy, intimacy, and most of its components (β = .135 and .121). In contrast, this student had lower preoccupied attachment (β = −.144). The student with higher maternal education was also higher in self-efficacy (β = .077). The Hong Kong student was lower than was the Mainland Chinese student in self-efficacy belief, secure attachment, dismissive attachment, intimacy, and most of its components. However, the Hong Kong student was higher in fearful attachment than was the Mainland counterpart (β = .095). The fan club member was higher in secure attachment and lower in preoccupied attachment than was the nonmember (β = .074 and −.073).

Concerning idolizing, background characteristics showed some differential effects due to the region and fan club membership. Generally, the Hong Kong student was significantly lower in idolizing than was the Chinese student (β = −.129). Nevertheless, the regional difference was insignificant in the early adolescent (β = −.041). Similarly, while the fan club member was generally and significantly higher in idolizing, the Hong Kong member did not exhibit a significant difference (β = .094).

Concerning idol glorifying, the gender, region, and fan club membership displayed some differentials among background characteristics. Gender made a significant difference in idol glorifying only in the older adolescent, such that the female student was higher than was the male (β = −.101). While the Hong Kong student was generally and significantly lower in idol glorifying, this regional difference was not significant in the early adolescent student. The fan club member was generally higher in idol glorifying. Nevertheless, the difference due to membership was not significant in Hong Kong (β = .022).

Concerning idol prizing, regional differences showed some differentials between the early adolescent and older adolescent. Accordingly, the older Hong Kong adolescent had significantly lower idol prizing than did the older Mainland adolescent (β = −.105). However, the younger Hong Kong adolescent showed higher idolizing than did the younger Mainland adolescent (β = .046). Hence, age made a difference in the region effect on idol prizing. Neither the region nor age made a significant difference in idol prizing.

Concerning idol modeling, the region exhibited some differentials across background characteristics. While gender difference was significant in the older student and Mainland student such that the female had lower idol modeling than did the male, the difference was insignificant in the early adolescent and Hong Kong student. In addition, the regional difference in idol modeling was greater in the male student and early adolescent than in the female student and older adolescent. Generally, nevertheless, the Hong Kong student was lower in idol modeling than was the Mainland student (β = −.200). While the fan club member was generally higher in idol modeling, the membership difference was insignificant in the male student, early adolescent, and Hong Kong Chinese.

Concerning idol romanticizing, differences due to the gender, region, and fan club membership manifested differentials across background characteristics. Generally, the female student was higher in idol romanticizing than was the male student ($\beta = .052$). Nevertheless, the Hong Kong female student was lower than was the Hong Kong male student in idol romanticizing, albeit insignificantly ($\beta = -.102$). The Hong Kong student was generally higher in idol romanticizing ($\beta = .090$). However, the regional difference was insignificant in the older adolescent ($\beta = -.004$). The fan club member was generally higher in idol romanticizing than was the nonmember ($\beta = .116$). However, the difference was insignificant and trivial in the male student ($\beta = .042$).

Concerning idol idealizing, difference due to fan club membership exhibited differentials across background characteristics. Generally, the member was higher in idol idealizing ($\beta = .095$). Nevertheless, the membership difference was smaller in the male student and Hong Kong student ($\beta = .088$ and $.067$).

Concerning idol commodifying, differences owing to the region, gender, paternal education, and fan club membership manifested some differentials across background characteristics. Notably, the female displayed significantly higher idol commodifying in Hong Kong ($\beta = .177$). Likewise, paternal education manifested a significant positive effect on idol commodifying only in Hong Kong ($\beta = .141$). Generally, the fan club member was significantly higher in idol commodifying than was the nonmember ($\beta = .211$). The membership difference was particularly greater in Hong Kong ($\beta = .249$). Meanwhile, the Hong Kong student was significantly higher than was the Mainland student in idol commodifying only when the student was an early adolescent ($\beta = .129$).

Concerning idol befriending, differences due to the region, age, gender, and fan club membership displayed some differentials across background characteristics. The female student was generally higher in idol befriending than was the male student ($\beta = .072$). The gender difference was particularly strong in the Hong Kong student ($\beta = .147$). However, the gender difference was weak in the Mainland Chinese student ($\beta = .051$). The older student was generally lower in idol befriending ($\beta = -.088$). The age difference was particularly great in the older adolescent and Mainland Chinese ($\beta = -.154$ and $-.142$). However, the older adolescent exhibited higher idol befriending than the early adolescent, albeit insignificantly ($\beta = .056$). The Hong Kong student was generally lower in idol befriending than was the Mainland student ($\beta = -.195$). This regional difference was particularly strong in the male student ($\beta = -.227$). The fan club member was generally higher in idol befriending than was the nonmember ($\beta = .127$). The membership difference was weaker in the Hong Kong student ($\beta = .105$).

Concerning idol faming, differences due to the region, gender, grade, and fan club membership manifested some differentials across background characteristics. Generally, the female student was lower in idol faming ($\beta = -.090$). However, the gender differences in the early adolescent and Hong Kong Chinese were very small ($\beta = -.025$ and $.011$). The school grade showed a significant negative effect on idol faming only in Hong Kong ($\beta = -.191$). The Hong Kong student was significantly lower in idol faming than was the Mainland student ($\beta = -.163$). Nevertheless, this regional difference was weaker in the early adolescent ($\beta = -.118$). The fan club member was generally higher in idol faming than was the nonmember ($\beta = .068$). However, the membership difference was very small, particularly in the male student and early adolescent (β = .055 and .044).

Concerning crediting, differences due to the region, school grade, and fan club membership displayed some differentials across background characteristics. Notably, the school grade had a significantly negative effect on idol crediting only in Hong Kong (β = −.235). The Hong Kong student was significantly lower in idol crediting than was the Mainland student (β = −.118). This regional difference was particularly strong in the male student (β = −.150). The fan club member was generally higher in idol crediting than was the nonmember (β = .055). Nevertheless, there was no membership difference in Hong Kong (β = −.016).

Concerning idol glamourizing, differences due to the region and fan club membership manifested some differentials across background characteristics. Generally, the Hong Kong student was significantly lower in idol glamourizing than was the Mainland student (β = −.107). Nevertheless, the difference was insignificant in the male student and early adolescent (β = −.077 and −.035). The fan club member was significantly higher in idol glamourizing than was the nonmember (β = .096). However, difference due to fan club membership was insignificant in the female and Hong Kong student (β = .051 and .000).

Concerning idol beautifying, differences due to gender, paternal education, and fan club membership displayed some differentials across background characteristics. The early female adolescent showed significantly higher idol beautifying than did the early male adolescent, whereas the older female adolescent displayed significantly lower idol beautifying than did the older male adolescent (β = .117 and −.107). Paternal education demonstrated a significant negative effect on idol beautifying in the male student, older adolescent, and Mainland Chinese (β = −.115, −.107, and −.074). In contrast, there was virtually no effect from paternal education on idol beautifying in the female student and early adolescent (β = .003 and .018). Generally, the fan club member was significantly higher in idol beautifying than was the nonmember (β = .060). The difference was not significant in the female student, older adolescent, and Hong Kong Chinese (β = .038, .048, and .009).

Concerning idol popularizing, differences due to gender, grade, and region maintained some differentials across background characteristics. The female student was significantly lower in idol popularizing than was the male student when the students were older or Mainland Chinese (β = −.096 and −.095). In contrast, the gender difference was insignificant in the early adolescent and Hong Kong Chinese (β = −.061 and −.055). The school grade generally showed a significant negative effect on idol popularizing (β = −.116). Nevertheless, the effect was insignificant in the female student, early adolescent, and Hong Kong Chinese (β = −.061, −.048, and −.092). The Hong Kong student was significantly higher in idol popularizing than was the Mainland counterpart (β = .200). The difference was particularly great in the early adolescent (β = .296).

Concerning idol personalizing, differences due to the age, school grade, region, and fan club membership exhibited some differentials across background characteristics. The female student was significantly higher than was the male student in idol personalizing when the students were early adolescents or Hong Kong Chinese ($\beta = .085$ and $.215$). In contrast, the gender difference was insignificant when the student was an older adolescent or Mainland Chinese ($\beta = .032$ and $.009$). The older girl displayed greater idol personalizing than the younger girl ($\beta = .139$). In contrast, the age effect was minimal in the male student ($\beta = .007$). Hence, age did not display a significant effect on idol personalizing generally ($\beta = .072$). The school grade manifested a significant positive effect on idol personalizing only in the male student ($\beta = .117$). Thus, the grade did not make a significant difference in idol personalizing generally ($\beta = .048$). The Hong Kong Chinese was generally lower in idol personalizing than was the Mainland Chinese ($\beta = -.227$). Such a regional difference was stronger in the male student ($\beta = -.318$). Generally, the fan club member was significantly higher in idol personalizing than was the nonmember ($\beta = .058$). The difference, nevertheless, was insignificant in the female student and Hong Kong Chinese ($\beta = .042$ and $.009$).

Concerning idol acceptance, differences due to the gender, region, grade, maternal school grade, and fan club membership displayed some variation across background characteristics. Generally, the female student held lower idol acceptance than did the male student ($\beta = -.066$). Although education generally did not have a significant effect on idol acceptance, it displayed a significant negative effect only in the male student ($\beta = -.129$). The maternal grade, in contrast, exhibited a significant positive effect on idol acceptance ($\beta = .077$). This effect was particularly significant in the Mainland student ($\beta = .086$). Generally, the Hong Kong student showed significantly lower idol acceptance than did the Mainland counterpart ($\beta = -.126$). This regional difference, nevertheless, was insignificant in the older adolescent ($\beta = -.042$). Generally, the fan club member was significantly higher in idol acceptance than was the nonmember ($\beta = .072$).

Concerning model acceptance, differences due to the gender, maternal grade, and region displayed some variation across background characteristics. Generally, the female student accepted the idol as a model less intensely than did the male student ($\beta = -.062$). Nevertheless, the gender difference was insignificant in the early adolescent and Hong Kong Chinese ($\beta = -.050$ and $-.042$). Maternal education displayed a significant positive effect on model acceptance ($\beta = .071$). The effect, nonetheless, was trivial in the male student, older adolescent, and Hong Kong Chinese ($\beta = .046, .047$, and $-.041$). Generally, the Hong Kong Chinese was significantly lower in model acceptance than was the Mainland Chinese ($\beta = -.144$). The regional difference was smaller in the older adolescent than in the younger ($\beta = -.082$).

Idolatry revealed in China

Analysis of survey data collected from 1,641 secondary school students in Mainland China and Hong Kong enables the enhancement of understanding about idolatry in youth. Such enhancement reveals the properties of idol choice, compensation, immaturity, gender variation, Chinese characteristics, and fandom in idolatry or its components.

Idolatry as celebrity worship

Idols chosen by Chinese secondary school students were predominantly celebrities (89.2%). Specifically, the idols were primarily stars (50.3%), entertainment figures (43.9%), historical figures (23.9%), political figures (12.6%), and athletic figures (6.0%). Moreover, idolizing displayed significant correlations with choice of an entertainment idol ($r = .141$, see Table 6.10), star idol ($r = .150$), and celebrity idol ($r = .053$). Celebrities and particularly entertainment or star figures are thereby the main target for idolatry. This is reasonably a result of the exposure, visibility, imaging, glamour, media creation, and even notoriety conferred on celebrities (Fraser and Brown 2002; Houran et al. 2005; Maltby et al. 2004a; North et al. 2005; Peng et al. 2010; Price et al. 2014; Reeves et al. 2012; Sivami et al. 2010). Similarly, celebrities have most likely counted as heroes (Madhavan and Crowell 2014). Celebrities also are prominent in education, advertising, media promotion, and socialization in general (Austin et al. 2008; Chiou et al. 2005). This is because of their remarkable social influence and persuasiveness (Hsiao 2004; Wen and Cui 2014). For youth, celebrities are easily recognizable and suitable to maintain parasocial relationships (Wen and Cui 2014). The youth is thereby susceptible to celebrities (Boon and Lomore 2001). This is thanks to celebrities' innovativeness and leadership in fashion (Law et al. 2000; Kawamura 2006). Hence, celebrities very likely become the target for idolatry (Chiou et al. 2005). Among celebrities, furthermore, stars are especially riveting, thanks to ingenious grooming and promotion by the entertainment industry (Lin and Lin 2007). Notably, stars have the qualities of talent, achievement, and fame (De Backer 2012; Hoegele et al. 2014). These qualities are exactly the target for idolizing, specifically crediting, faming, glorifying, prizing, and modeling. Similarly, entertainment is a basic criterion for idolatry (Maltby et al. 2004b; McCutcheon et al. 2003; Pang et al. 2010; Sheridan et al. 2007). Entertainers are thus favorites for idolatry.

Idolatry as compensation

Compensation between idolatry and other engagements is evident in China, involving both Mainland and Hong Kong Chinese. This is identifiable with inverse relationships between idolizing on the one hand and self-efficacy belief, secure attachment, and intimacy with the closest friend on the other. This generally applies to the components of idolizing as well as overall idolizing. The compensation theory thus suggests that idolatry originates and/or engenders deficiency in other engagements. This suggestion is consistent with existing findings about correlates, predictors, or outcomes of idolatry. Accordingly, deficiency dispositions predictive of idolatry are cognitive deficit, cognitive inflexibility, dissociation, narcissism, and psychopathy (Maltby et al. 2004;

McCutcheon et al. 2003; Moriarty 1992; Southard and Zeigler-Hill 2016). Furthermore, deficiency experiences predictive of idolatry are threat, peer conflict, illness, and loss (Moriarty 1992). The experiences have also been predictive of detachment from parents and intention to use pirated products (Giles and Maltby 2004; C. Wang et al. 2009). Moreover, deficiency feelings predictive of idolatry are boredom, anger, life dissatisfaction, self-disrespect, and self-ambiguity (Reeves et al. 2012; S. Ryu et al. 2007). Meanwhile, idolatry erodes such traits as creativity and critical thinking (Houran et al. 2005). Idolatry also foments such deficiency practices as aggression, compulsive and impulsive buying, and criminality (Greenwood 2007; Niu and Wang 2009; Reeves et al. 2012; Sheridan et al. 2007). Furthermore, idolatry engenders deficient consequences in feeling by weakening adjustment and satisfaction and increasing feelings of guilt (Moriarty 1992; Scharf and Levy 2015).

Compensation between idolatry and other engagements was greater in the female student, older adolescent, and Hong Kong Chinese than in the male student, early adolescent, and Mainland Chinese. The greater compensation or contrast in the female student than in the male student reflects her greater relational selectivity, identification, affiliation, and maintenance (Dunkel et al. 2016; Galambos et al. 2009; Zupancic et al. 2014). That is, young girls are more faithful and careful in relationships, and thereby differentiate between various relationships. Hence, the female youth is more socially sensitive, investigative, committed, and concerned with group membership than is the male youth (Catalano et al. 2003; Cattarello 2000; Lessard et al. 2011; Lim 1995; Newman et al. 2007; Tokar et al. 2007; Weems et al. 2002). Behaviorally, the female youth is higher than the male youth in social comparison (Morrison et al. 2004). Meanwhile, the greater compensation in the older youth reflects cognitive development, which facilitates differentiation and identification (Gibbs et al. 2007; Owens et al. 2005). Consistent with cognitive development with age is growth in the traits of intelligence, knowledge, competence, and morality and moral reasoning (Barrett 2007; Krauss et al. 2014; Markoulis and Valanides 1997; Tinsley and Spencer 2010; van Goethem et al. 2012). Prejudice and discrimination also grow with age (Barrett 2007). Behaviorally, the older youth is more socially aware (Pinquart and Pfeiffer 2013). Likewise, increase in compensation with education reflects cognitive development, which fosters differentiation (Furnham-Diggory 1992). With education, the youth displays growth in the traits of intelligence, knowledge, competence, and curiosity (Bidwell et al. 1996; Brouwers et al. 2006; Crystal and DeBell 2002; Yi et al. 2004). Education increases such practices as elaboration and social comparison (Jakoubek and Swenson 1993; Schutz et al. 2002). The Hong Kong Chinese exhibits greater compensation than does the Mainland Chinese, and this is attributable to some regional differences. Accordingly, the Hong Kong youth has such characteristics as social comparison and taking multiple perspectives (D. Chan 2008; Fairbrother 2003). In contrast, the Mainland Chinese youth displays such characteristics as goal alignment, social connectedness, and having diverse relations (Keller and Loewenstein 2011; Liu et al. 2005). These differences in sensitivity, differentiation, elaboration, comparison, and discrimination as opposed to maintaining consistency and connectedness would explain differentials in compensation among students of different genders, ages, education levels, and regions.

Idol modeling, befriending, and personalizing as spillover

There are some exceptions to idol modeling, befriending, and personalizing, which are components of idolizing. Specifically, idol modeling exhibited positive correlations with self-efficacy and secure attachment, idol befriending showed a positive correlation with secure attachment, and idol personalizing indicated positive correlations with self-efficacy, secure attachment, and intimacy. These correlations imply spillover between these idolizing components and other engagements. Such spillover is favorable because of the intrinsic and extrinsic merits of self-efficacy, attachment security, and intimacy (Cotterell 2007; Fosco and Feinberg 2015; Hand et al. 2013; Henderson et al. 2009; Hirschi 2009; Vivona 2000). Meanwhile, idol modeling, befriending, and personalizing have their intrinsic and extrinsic merits, too. Idol modeling involves identification, learning, and emulation, which can be fundamental to the development of leadership, endurance, talents, and socializing (Bowers et al. 2016; Fraser and Brown 2002; Lempers and Clark-Lempers 1993; Raviv et al. 1996; C. Wang et al. 2009).

Idol modeling is beneficial on a number of grounds. Most obviously, idol modeling means becoming similar to the idol, including his or her talents and merits (Calvert et al. 2004; Greene and Adams-Price 1990; Lindenberg et al. 2011; S. Ryu et al. 2007; C. Wang et al. 2009). Idol modeling also sustains the motive of self-expansion in identifying idols similar to oneself to magnify one's significance (Huang and Mitchell 2014). The learning component of idol modeling generally is creditable for its contribution to problem solving, skill development, and eventually satisfaction (Kasen et al. 2004; Lee and Fortune 2013). Intrinsically, idol modeling is necessary as a way of role modeling or taking (Girsh 2014; Buxton 1983; Stevens 2010). Hence, idol modeling realizes teleological and consequentialist merits. Modeling in general also has a favorable, prosocial basis to champion its deontological or formalist value (Wang 1994).

Idol befriending has a number of favorable properties to champion its favorable spillover. By nature, idol befriending means trusting the idol and believing in his or her sociability, friendliness, and goodwill, which is conducive to a sense of security (Giles and Maltby 2004; Gleason et al. 2017; Pleiss and Feldhusen 1995). Befriending, without romantic or erotic overtones, would thereby be helpful to cognitive or intellectual development (Adams-Price and Greene 1990). More than providing security, befriending is likely to realize the benefits of friendship in achieving attachment, acceptance, intimacy, reciprocity, popularity, and normative development (Espelage et al. 2007; Hartup 1996; Light and Dishion 2007; Pellegrini and Blatchford 2000; Seibert and Kerns 2009).

A cognitive credit of befriending is equilibration or reconciliation of cognitive conflict through understanding and balancing ideas between oneself and friends (Pellegrini and Blatchford 2000). Instrumentally, befriending is likely to contribute to belongingness, self-esteem, and reduction in loneliness (Brendgen et al. 2000; Falci and McNeely 2009; Wu and Wong 2013; Zysberg 2012). Furthermore, befriending has the potential to raise moral and prosocial behavior and prevent problem behavior, such as school dropout and theft (Elliott et al. 2006; McCarthy et al. 2004; Staff and Kraeger 2008; Wu and Wong 2013). Befriending is also likely to foster attachment to or affiliation with school (Benson 2007; Moody and White 2003; Wu and Wong 2013). The contribution of friendship, according to the utilitarian view, is its provision of happiness and acceptance to satisfy interests (Grunebaum 2003). Friendship is also favorable in its realization of personal choice, according to the libertarian view (Grunebaum 2003). Moreover, friendship rests on the basis of secure attachment, notably manifested in parental attachment (Bagwell and Schmidt 2011; Parade et al. 2010). Well-being as opposed to anxiety and depression contributes to friendship (Parade et al. 2010; van Zalk et al. 2010). These are favorable deontological bases for friendship. Hence, friendship is both extrinsically and intrinsically valuable. Moreover, befriending is valuable through trusting, which enhances competence, vitality, self-esteem, and identity commitment and achievement (Crystal and DeBell 2002; Hoegh and Bourgeois 2002; Meeus et al. 2002). In addition, trust prevents depression (M. Wu et al. 2010). Trust is also favorable in view of its contribution to secure attachment, morality, and citizenship (Crystal and DeBell 2002; Hoegh and Bourgeois 2002; King 2007). This may result from the contribution of trust to friendship and care reception (Meeus et al. 2002; Nucci 2006). Furthermore, trust is valuable in light of its contribution to volunteering and moral behavior (King and Furrow 2004; Marzana et al. 2012). Trust prevents doping, alcoholism, and school dropout (Dufur et al. 2013; Kirk 2009). The merit of trust, according to the communitarian view, rests on the human desire for and benefit from community, friendship, cooperation, and sharing (Abascal 2015). This means that trust is beneficial due to its contribution of need fulfillment. Hence, idol befriending, by holding trust and friendship, is justifiably favorable both personally and socially.

Idol personalizing is favorable in realizing personal choice or autonomy (Giles and Maltby 2004; Greene and Adams-Price 1990). Choice and autonomy are vital for this signification of identity or self (Yeh and Yan 2006). All these are pertinent to fundamental needs in youth development (McElhaney et al. 2009). Accordingly, individuation and detachment are essential to goal setting and attachment (McElhaney et al. 2009; Pfeiffer and Pinquart 2012; Yeh and Yan 2006). Autonomy demonstrates a contribution to happiness, self-esteem, and social skill (Yeh and Yang 2006). In addition, autonomy inhibits externalizing and internalizing problems and noncompliance (Kasen et al. 2004; Yeh and Yang 2006). Meanwhile, autonomy has a basis in secure attachment and goal engagement (McElhaney et al. 2009; Pfeiffer and Pinquart 2012). As such, safety and social support in the environment are contributors to autonomy (Krauss et al. 2014).

Furthermore, school connectedness and agentic engagement sustain autonomy (Krauss et al. 2014; Schenke et al. 2015). Autonomy thus has favorable bases as well as consequences. Idol personalizing, with its realization of autonomy, thus secures deontological, teleological, and consequentialist bases for its merit.

Spillover between idol modeling, idol befriending, and idol personalizing on the one hand and self-efficacy on the other hand, however, did not happen in the Hong Kong Chinese. In such a student, instead, compensation prevailed. This reflects the cultural characteristics of concentration as opposed to curiosity and holding multiple perspectives in Hong Kong youth (Fairbrother 2003). As such, given high self-efficacy, the need for idol modeling, befriending, and personalizing would be low and vice versa.

Idol popularizing and befriending as immaturity

Two components of idolatry, idol popularizing and befriending, showed a significant decline with age and education. In the first place, age and education signify maturity (Baer 2002; Furnham-Diggory 1992; Monahan et al. 2013; Owens et al. 2005; Winters et al. 1995). As such, older age and higher education mean greater learning, knowledge, capability, articulation, exploration, reflection, cultivation, cooperation, cognitive complexity, and experiential diversity (Furnham-Diggory 1992; Hwang 2013). Meanwhile, idol popularizing and befriending tend to represent immaturity. On the one hand, idol popularizing involves conforming and following as opposed to individuation, differentiation, and creativity (He and Feng 2002; Lindenberg et al. 2011). Conformity shows a decline with education, moral reasoning, verbal ability, creativity, and intellectual quality (Rest et al. 1999; Wilder et al. 2000). On the other hand, idol befriending involves gullibility, unwariness, and lack of deliberation or critical thinking (Buxton 1983; Garratt 1984; Houran et al. 2005; McCutcheon et al. 2003). Meanwhile, critical thinking rests on age and education (Giancarlo and Facione 2001; Kramer and Melchoir 1990; Spaulding and Kleiner 1992). Critical thinking also notably increases with verbal ability, particularly improved vocabulary (Kramer and Melchoir 1990). Moreover, developmental programs promoting thinking, learning, challenging, curiosity, brainstorming, differentiation, questioning, role playing, and others increase critical thinking (Bensley and Haynes 1995; Blinde 1995; Brookfield 1987; Browne 2000; Donay and Lephardt 1993; Johnson and Johnson 1993; Kaplan and Kies 1994; McEwen 1994; Misra 1997; Pithers and Soden 2000; Reed and Kromrey 2001; Shepelak 1996; Sparapani 1998; Walkner and Finney 1999). Conversely, being uncritical in idol befriending registers immaturity.

The immature property of idol popularizing and befriending was greater in the male student than in the female student. This means that the maturation effect is stronger in the male youth than in the female youth, such that the maturing male youth reduces idol popularizing and befriending more intensely than the maturing female youth. In other words, maturation or age and education is more influential or valuable in the male youth than in the female youth. This echoes the greater valuation of academic study, employment, and earnings in the male youth than in the female youth (Eccles 1985; Ovadia 2001; Thompson and Petrovic 2009). Similarly, the male youth finds greater academic benefits than does the female youth (Becker and Hecken 2009). Valuation of or sensitivity to maturation is also a greater concern for the male youth than the female youth for social status and resource acquisition (Dunkel et al. 2016; Galambos et al. 2009; Toro-Morn and Sprecher 2003).

Idol romanticizing as maturity

In contrast with the immature property of idol popularizing and befriending, idol romanticizing represented maturity with a positive correlation with age, particularly in the Mainland Chinese. This maturation effect is evident in the increase in romantic orientation and practice with age (Cavanagh 2011; Halpern et al. 2005; McCarthy and Casey 2008; Pinquart and Pfeiffer 2013). The increase also reflects the growth of need and favor for intimacy and romantic love with age (Giordano et al. 2006; Gummerum and Keller 2008; Sumter et al. 2013; Zimmer-Gembeck et al. 2012). Moreover, the pronounced maturation effect in Mainland China reflects the importance of maturation, adulthood, and marriage in Mainland China and its youth (Liao et al. 2011; Liu et al. 2005; Zhang and Thomas 1994). By contrast, there was no maturation effect of idol romanticizing in Hong Kong, where youth and identity moratorium rather than maturation are favorable (Kam 2012). That is, concern for marriage and romantic love would not substantially increase with age during secondary schooling in Hong Kong. Instead, the concern is likely to increase after secondary schooling there.

Idolatry as a gendered expression

The male student and female student exhibited different forms of idolatry. Specifically, the male student manifested greater idol faming and idol and model acceptance than did the female student. Moreover, the male student's idol was more likely to be a Western idol, athletic idol, military idol, business idol, or historical idol than was the female student's idol. These features appear to be masculine. Notably, masculinity is defined as being distinguished, famous, and having a clearly defined position in society (Korobov 2004). Moreover, such idolatry reflects the male youth's higher assertiveness, competitiveness, entrepreneurship, mammonism, manipulativeness, patriotism, and broad-based knowledge pursuit (Barrett 2007; Ekstrom and Ostman 2013; Flanagan and Campbell 2003; Lessard et al. 2011; Liu et al. 2009; Lusardi et al. 2010; Niemi et al. 2000; Ovadia 2001; Schmitt-Redermund and Vondracek 2002; Walstad et al. 2010). The male youth also shows higher favor for competition and politics than does the female youth (Lucas and Sherry 2004; Matthews and Howell 2006). Behaviorally, the male youth has more exercise, gaming, and sport participation than has the female youth (Chen et al. 2007; Cradock et al. 2009;

Garcia et al. 2016; Glanville et al. 2008; Lucas and Sherry 2004; Morrison et al. 2004). These differences possibly stem from evolutionary mechanisms to assign acquisitive qualities to the male (Dunkel et al. 2016; Galambos et al. 2009). Such assignment, furthermore, receives reinforcement from socialization or sociocultural processes (Sumter et al. 2013; Zupancic et al. 2014).

In contrast, idol romanticizing and befriending were higher in the female Chinese than in the male counterpart, reflecting its feminine basis. This notably echoes existing findings about the female edge in romanticizing (Adams-Price and Greene 1990; Argyle 1994; Greene and Adams-Price 1990). Meanwhile, the female youth is higher in the traits of agreeableness, dependability, gratitude, and kindness (Hill and Rojewski 1999; Liu et al. 2009; Shimai et al. 2006). Moreover, the female gender breeds such attitudes as favor especially romance, attachment (especially romantic attachment), appreciation, compliance, liking, tolerance, susceptibility, support, and trust (Awang et al. 2013; Calvert et al. 2004; Ekstrom and Ostman 2013; Feiring 1995; Flanagan and Campbell 2003; Hooghe et al. 2015; Jones and Watt 1999; Shimai et al. 2006; Unger et al. 2001; Watt et al. 2017). The female gender also espouses the practices of body idealization, conformity, consumption, dating, and romantic involvement (Cavanagh 2007; Dunn et al. 2010; Feiring 1995; Furman and Winkles 2010; McCarthy and Cassy 2008; Wilder et al. 2000). All these properties are compatible with idol prizing, romanticizing, commodifying, idealizing, and/or befriending. Conversely, the female gender erodes the traits of rebelliousness, competitiveness, thrift, and realism (Bleich et al. 1991; Flanagan and Campbell 2003; Ovadia 2001; Power and Khmelkov 1999; Tokar et al. 2007; Zhang 2008). Moreover, the female gender diminishes favorable attitudes toward challenging, competition, and callousness (Lessard et al. 2011; Lucas and Sherry 2004). Behaviorally, the female youth is lower than the male in disrespect, discriminating, annoying, protest, violence, and conflict with others (De Bruyn et al. 2003; Forman 2001; Rudasill et al. 2014; Strohschein and Matthew 2015; Swank 2012). The erosion of these properties enables idol prizing.

The female student shows certain preferences for idols' features, including the female idol, entertainment idol, star idol, and literary idol, as compared with the male student. In the first place, preference of the same-sex idol is evident. This indicates that the idol is more likely to count as a friend rather than a lover of the opposite sex to meet the needs for validation and modeling for adaptation (Feldman and Wentzel 1995; Lempers and Clark-Lempers 1993). Moreover, the preferences reflect the characteristics of the female youth in verbal ability and orientation, romantic orientation, and beauty appreciation (Bodovski 2010; Furman and Winkles 2010; Feiring 1995; Gottfried 2013; McCarthy and Casey 2008; Shimai et al. 2006; Tanskanen 2016). Conversely, the female youth dislikes callousness and realism more than does the male youth (Lessard et al. 2011; Tokar et al. 2007; Zhang 2008).

The female student displayed lower idol glorifying (including glamourizing, faming, and crediting) and idol beautifying than did the male student, particularly when the students were older adolescents. In the first place, the lower glorifying in the female student reflects the female youth's lower favor for the partner's attractiveness and higher valuation of equality (Ekstrom and Ostman 2013; Ovadia 2001; Toro-Morn and Sprecher 2003). It is traceable to evolutionary processes underlying gender differences (Dunkel et al. 2016; Galambos et al. 2009). Such evolutionarily based gender differences increase with age or maturity (Monahan et al. 2013).

The female student showed less idol modeling than did the male student, particularly when the students were Mainland Chinese. Traditionally, this reflects the female youth's lower curiosity and identification with others (Froiland et al. 2015; Greene and Adams-Price 1990). This tradition would be stronger in Mainland China, which is rather traditional (Wang and Zhu 1996).

The female student revealed greater idol personalizing than did the male student, particularly when the students were Hong Kong Chinese. This is obviously due to the greater favor for personalization and self-expression in the female youth than in the male youth (Adams-Price and Greene 1990; Cash and Conway 1997; Lim 1995). Such individualistic female properties would be particularly acceptable and thus prominent in Hong Kong, where individualization prevails (Lai and Begram 2003).

Idolatry as a Chinese characteristic

Idolatry, including idolizing and acceptance, was greater in the Mainland Chinese than in the Hong Kong Chinese. As such, idolatry characterizes Mainland China more than Hong Kong. A prominent difference between Mainland China and Hong Kong is the latter's higher Westernization, globalization, and internationalization (K. Cheung 2015; Chui and Chan 2012; Kuah-Pearce and Fong 2010). Such tendencies are likely to diminish cultural concerns for norms, morality, and trust in authority (Ikels 1989; H. Ng 2015). By contrast, Mainland China has the cultural characteristics of atheism, nonreligiosity, hierarchism, conformity, obedience, deference, respect, and normativity (Cheung and Pomerantz 2011; Cui et al. 2016; King and Roeser 2009; Liao et al. 2011; Naftali 2009; Nelson and Barry 2005; Peng et al. 2015; Zhan and Ning 2004; Zhang 2003; Zhu 2006). Furthermore, the polity and education in Mainland China encourage character, moral, civic, and political education, which emphasize conformity, normativity, nationalism, and patriotism (Lawrence 2000; Lee and Ho 2005; Wu 2003; Zhan and Ning 2004; Zhang 2003; Zhu 2006). Hence, Mainland China espouses the culture of idolatry for youth (He 2006; Qi and Tang 2004). Idols importantly serve as exemplars, motivators, teachers, and paragons to boost youths' talents, character, confidence, courage, erudition, patriotism, achievement, and even beauty in Mainland China (He 2006).

Moreover, idol features were more diverse in Mainland Chinese students than in Hong Kong Chinese students. Accordingly, the Mainland Chinese student was more likely to adore the luminary idol, historical idol, Western idol, athletic idol, academic idol, literary idol, political idol, scientist idol, familial idol, peer idol, and noncelebrity idol than was the Hong Kong student. This echoes the greater emphasis on patriotic and history education and the family in Mainland China (Luk 2001; Wang 2008). In contrast, the Hong Kong student was more likely to worship an entertainment idol, star idol, altruistic idol, idealistic idol, Japanese idol, female idol, or celebrity idol than was the Mainland Chinese student. The scope of idol features was hence narrower in Hong Kong than in Mainland China. This reflects the service industry and its mediatization in Hong Kong to popularize celebrity idols (K. Cheung 2015; Lee and Ting 2015).

Idolatry as fandom

Idolatry is associated with fandom, in view of the positive correlation with fan club membership. The correlation was stronger in idol commodifying, befriending, and romanticizing than in the other components of idolatry. There are also significant positive correlations between fan club membership and the choice of entertainment idol and star idol. Idolatry involving such idols is clearly associated with fandom (End et al. 2002; Ferris 2001). Furthermore, fandom buttresses idolatry as a social activity through fan clubs and their social integration function (Turner and Scherman 1996). Idolatry in this sense is a social or even socially constructed activity to maintain group solidarity and identity (Reijnders et al. 2007; Wang 1994). That is, idolatry in the context of a fan club is more than parasocial interaction. Moreover, personal entertainment through fans' idolatry is a social property (Maltby et al. 2004b; Peng et al. 2015; Sheridan et al. 2007). Furthermore, such fandom-driven idolatry may represent social obsession (McCutcheon et al. 2002). In contrast, there are significant negative correlations between fan club membership and the choice of historical idol and luminary idol. Obviously, historical and luminary idols are not the target for the formation of fan clubs.

The association between fan club membership and idolizing, particularly idol glorifying, idealizing, crediting, glamourizing, beautifying, and personalizing, was particularly weak in Hong Kong. This tends to reflect the weak organizing, grouping, and collective power and orientation there (Chan 2001). The weakness is due to dilution from the plurality and diversity of groups and clubs (Forestier and Crossley 2015; Ma 2011b; Oksanen 2011).

Summary

Youth idolatry, as implied in the analysis of survey data collected in Mainland China and Hong Kong, manifests the primary property of compensation with other engagements, including self-efficacy, intimacy, and secure attachment. Compensation suggests that idolatry results from inadequacy in other engagements or impedes other engagements. Furthermore, compensation is consonant with views that idolatry results from problems in identity, self, attachment, and cognitive development (Cole and Leats 1999; Jenson 1992; Maltby et al. 2004b; McCutcheon et al. 2003; Noser and Zeigler-Hill 2014; Reeves et al. 2012; Seiffge-Krenke 1997). Hence, personal emptiness, egocentrism, narcissism, depression, and uncertainty on the one hand and relational insecurity, isolation, and weakness on the other are precursors to idolatry. In addition, the compensation thesis is compatible with the contributions of idolatry to dissatisfaction, maladjustment, guilty feelings, aggression, compulsive and impulsive buying, sexual permissiveness, and even criminality (Greenwood 2007; Moriarty 1992; Niu and Wang 2009; Reeves et al. 2012; Scharf and Levy 2015; Sheridan et al. 2007). Furthermore, the thesis is also compatible with the negative effects of idolatry on creativity and critical thinking (Houran et al. 2005). That is, idolatry displaces well-being and good practices.

An exception is the idolizing component of idol modeling or emulation, which displayed spillover with other engagements in the Chinese youth. Idol modeling thus rests on and/or buttresses self-efficacy, intimacy, and secure attachment. This reflects self-expansion as a specific basis for the spillover (Huang and Mitchell 2014). Accordingly, modeling after the idol represents the expansion of the self to the idol and vice versa. Such a modeling or spillover thesis is compatible with the contributions of modeling or learning to skill, performance, and satisfaction (Kasen el al. 2004; Lee and Fortune 2013). Hence, idol modeling is disparate from idolatry in general.

Glossary

Absorption-addiction idolatry (AAI)   describes an irrational, obsessive idolatry that involves a full commitment of available perceptual, motoric, imaginative, and ideational resources to form a unified representation of idolized figures.

Attachment   refers to the bond between an infant and a caregiver. It influences one's ability to form stable relationships throughout life.

Attachment styles   reflect beliefs in the internal mental working models crucial for social interaction and relationship building. According to attachment theory, four distinct styles of attachment have been identified in adults: secure, anxious-preoccupied, dismissive-avoidant, and fearful-avoidant.

Attributes-focused idol worship 特质为本型偶像崇拜   is a kind of idolatry that is represented by the fan's admiration of and identification with desirable and imitable attributes of different favored idols.

Beautifying of the idol   means regarding the idol as a beautiful woman, handsome man, or as physically attractive and worthy of adoring or appreciating.

Befriending of the idol   means regarding the idol as a friend, typically with warmth, sociability, and amity, to maintain contact, conversation, interaction, friendship, attachment, and even intimacy.

Celebrity worship 名人崇拜   means to adore or idolize famous people, whether at present or in the past.

Commodifying of the idol   means subscribing to the idol's materials, typically commodities for possession, consumption, maintaining contact, and/or adoring.

Compatibility perspective of idol worship 偶像崇拜相容论   suggests that idol worship includes compatible parasocial and social interactions in idolatrous behaviors such that it complements one's self-development.

Compensatory perspective of idol worship 偶像崇拜补偿论   regards idol worshippers as being absorbed, addicted, obsessive individuals who lack meaningful relationships.

Crediting of the idol   means acclaiming the idol's success, talent, and/or other good features for admiring or esteeming.

Faming of the idol   means regarding the idol as famous. In other words, faming means honoring or acclaiming the idol.

Fan 粉丝   is either an enthusiastic devotee (as of a sport or a performing art) usually as a spectator or an ardent admirer or enthusiast (as of a celebrity or a pursuit).

Fandom   refers to the state or attitude of being a fan.

Glamourizing of the idol   means to treat the idol as charming and thus induce indulgence.

Identification-emulation idolatry (IEI)   describes a rational and nonobsessive idolatry that features identification with and emulation of enhanced or idealized attributes of idolized figures.

Identity achievement   involves exploration of and eventual commitment to goals about one's career, sexuality and marriage, family, religion and beliefs, community, and political involvement.

Idol 偶像   is a representation or symbol of an object of worship.

Idolatry 偶像崇拜   refers to worship of a physical image, such as a statue, an icon, or a real person.

Idol figure 偶像人物   is typically a celebrity, a hero/heroine, or a luminary figure.

Idol worship 偶像崇拜   literally means worship of a physical image or a figure other than a Supreme Being for gaining power, protection, or fantasized intimacy. It is often used interchangeably with *idolatry*.

Intimacy   refers to a close, familiar, and usually affectionate or loving personal relationship with another person or a group.

Modeling of the idol   means setting the idol as a model for learning, emulation, and/or identifying.

Personalizing the idol   means maintaining the idol as a fit to oneself for cherishing, due to commitment to personal choice.

Person-focused idol worship 人物为本型偶像崇拜   is a kind of idolatry that features the fan's admiration or mystification of a particular idol as possessing all desirable attributes.

Popularizing the idol   means regarding the idol as popular, notably among significant others.

Role model learning   means to encourage students to develop their talents and learn new skills.

Romanticizing of the idol   means attributing romance and lovability to the idol for loving or infatuation.

Self-efficacy   refers to belief in one's own ability to achieve or tackle problems generally.

Tri-star idols   include pop stars, movie stars, sport stars, and the like.

Notes

1 Idol worship and related concepts

1 Wei Jie (衛玠285–314), Wei and Jin dynasty (魏晉朝代), is also famous for his philosophical viewpoints.

2 Theories and perspectives of idol worship

1 Andy Lau (劉德華1961–), a Hong Kong actor, singer, lyricist, and film producer, has been one of Hong Kong's most commercially successful film actors since the mid-1980s, performing in more than 160 films while maintaining a successful singing career. In the 1990s, the media named him one of the Four Heavenly Kings of Cantopop (四大天王).

2 Li Yuchun (Chinese: 李宇春, 1984–), also known as Chris Lee, is a Chinese singer, songwriter, and actress. She debuted her singing career by winning the Chinese singing contest *Supergirl* in 2005. The next year she released her debut album, *The Queen and the Dreams*. She is often referred to as the mother of the unisex look in China, where she has achieved success.

3 Lei Feng (雷鋒 1940–1962) was a driver for an army unit in northeastern China and reportedly did many "good things" for friends or strangers before he died in active service. He is considered a model soldier and citizen for the new China. He is often quoted as saying: "Life is limited and should be used for unlimited service."

4 Top leaders in socialist China praised Lei Feng to promote him as a public model. Mao Ze Dong's slogan "Learn from Comrade Lei Feng" (向雷鋒同志學習) was once painted on every school in China.

3 Comparing and verifying absorption-addiction idolatry and identification-emulation idolatry

1 Faye Wong (1969–), a Chinese singer-songwriter and actress, is often called the "diva" (天后; Heavenly Queen) among Chinese singers. In 2000, the *Guinness Book of World Records* recognized her as the best-selling Cantopop female singer. She moved to Hong Kong from Beijing in 1987 and quickly gained public attention by singing in Cantonese and Mandarin.

2 November 11 (Double 11) is Bachelor's Day, a day when young people hold parties to help single people meet, become engaged, or simply have fun. Alibaba held its first Double 11 Shopping Festival in 2009 on Taobao.com. It has quickly become a symbol for e-commerce in China: https://www.chinainternetwatch.com/tag/double-11/#ixzz58z5HoOMD.

3 Louis Cha Leung-yung, GBM, OBE, better known by his pen name, Jin Yong, is a Chinese wuxia novelist and essayist who cofounded and served as first editor in chief of the Hong Kong daily newspaper *Ming Pao* in 1959.

References

Aaker, Jennifer L., Emily N. Garbinsky, and Kathleen D. Voh. 2012. "Cultivating Admiration in Brands: Warmth, Competence, and Landing in the Golden Quadrant." *Journal of Consumer Psychology* 22(2):191–194.

Abada, Teresa, Feng Hou, and Bali Ram. 2007. "Racially Mixed Neighborhoods, Perceived Neighborhood Social Cohesion, and Adolescent Health in Canada." *Social Science & Medicine* 65:2004–2017.

Abascal, M. 2015. "Love thy Neighbor: Ethnoracial Diversity and Trust Reexamined." *American Journal of Sociology* 121(3):622–782.

Aberg, Yvonne, and Peter Hedstrom. 2011. "Youth Unemployment: A Self-reinforcing Process?" pp. 201–226 in *Analytical Sociology and Social Mechanisms*, edited by Pierre Demeulenaere. Cambridge, UK: Cambridge University Press.

Abraham, L., M. Potegal, and S. Miller. 1983. "Evidence for Caudate Nucleus Involvement in an Egocentric Spatial Task: Return from Passive Transport." *Physiological Psychology* 11(1):11–17.

Adams, Gerald R., Bruce A. Ryan, and Leo Keating. 2000. "Family Relationships, Academic Environments, and Psychosocial Development during the University Experience: A Longitudinal Investigation." *Journal of Adolescent Research* 15(1):99–122.

Adams, G. R., and J. A. Shea. 1979. "The Relationship between Identity Status, Locus of Control, and Ego Development." *Journal of Youth and Adolescence* 8(1):81–89.

Adams, G. R., J. H. Ryan, J. J. Hoffman, W. R. Dobson, and E. C. Neilsen. 1985. "Ego Identity Status, Conformity Behavior, and Personality in Late Adolescence." *Journal of Personality and Social Psychology* 47:1091–1104.

Adams, Gerald R. 1985. "Identity and Political Socialization." *New Directions for Child Development* 30:61–77.

Adams-Price, Carolyn, and A. L. Greene. 1990. "Secondary Attachments and Adolescent Self Concept." *Sex Roles* 22(3/4):187–198.

Adler, Patricia A., and Peter Adler. 1999. "Transience and the Postmodern Self: The Geographic Mobility of Resort Workers." *Sociological Quarterly* 40(1):31–58.

Agnew, Robert. 2002. "Experienced, Vicarious, and Anticipated Strain: An Exploratory Study on Physical Victimization and Delinquency." *Justice Quarterly* 19(4):603–632.

Ainsworth, M. S. 1985. "Attachment across the Lifespan." *Bulletin of the New York Academy of Medicine* 61:792–812.

Ainsworth, M. S. 1989. "Attachments Beyond Infancy." *American Psychologist* 44(4):709.

Alexander, J. C. 2010. "The Celebrity-Icon." *Cultural Sociology* 4(3):323–336.

Alfeld-Liro, Corinne, and Carol K. Sigelman. 1998. "Sex Differences in Self-concept and Symptoms of Depression during the Transition to College." *Journal of Youth & Adolescence* 27(2):219–244.

Algoe, Sara B., and Jonathan Haidt. 2009. "Witnessing Excellence in Action: The Other-Praising Emotions of Elevation, Gratitude, and Admiration." *Journal of Positive Psychology* 4(2):105–127.

Al-krenawi, Alean, John R. Graham, Fakir Al Gharaibeh. 2011. "A Comparison Study of Psychological, Family Function Marital and Life Satisfactions of Polygamous and Monogamous Women in Jordan." *Community Mental Health Journal* 47(5):594–602.

Allen, Steven G., Robert L. Clark, and Linda S. Ghent. 2005. "Phasing into Retirement." *Industrial & Labor Relations Review* 58(1):112–127.

Allison, Scott T., and George R. Goethals. 2016. "Hero Worship: The Elevation of the Human Spirit." *Journal for the Theory of Social Behaviour* 46(2):187–210.

Allport, G. W. 1950. "The Individual and His Religion." New York: MacMillan.

Allport, G. W., and J. M. Ross. 1967. "Personal Religious Orientation and Prejudice." *Journal of Personality and Social Psychology* 5:432–433.

Almgren, Gunnar, Maya Magarati, and Liz Mogford. 2009. "Examining the Influences of Gender, Race, Ethnicity, and Social Capital on the Subjective Health of Adolescents." *Journal of Adolescence* 32:109–133.

Alsord, Sarah H., L. David Brown, and Christine W. Letts. 2004. "Social Entrepreneurship and Societal Transformation: An Exploratory Study." *Journal of Applied Behavioral Science* 40(3):260–282.

Anderson-Butcher, Dawn, Aidyn L. Iachini, and Anthony J. Amorose. 2008. "Initially Reliability and Validity of the Perceived Social Competence Scale." *Research on Social Work Practice* 18(1):47–54.

Appleton, Simon, and Lina Song. 2008. "Life Satisfaction in Urban China: Components and Determinants." *World Development* 36(11):2335–2340.

Aquino, Karl, and Dan Freeman. 2009. "Moral Identity in Business Situations: A Social-cognitive Framework for Understanding Moral Functioning." pp. 375–395 in *Personality, Identity, and Character: Explorations in Moral Psychology*, edited by Darcin Narvaez and Daniel K. Lapsley. New York: Cambridge University Press.

Arbona, C., and T. G. Power. 2003. "Parental Attachment, Self-esteem, and Antisocial Behaviors among African American, European American, and Mexican American Adolescents." *Journal of Counseling Psychology* 50(1):40.

Ardichvili, Alexander. 2001. "Leadership Styles of Russian Entrepreneurs and Managers." *Journal of Developmental Entrepreneurship* 6(2):169–187.

Argyle, Michael. 1994. *The Psychology of Social Class*. London: Routledge.

Armitage, C. J., and P. R. Harris. 2006. "The Influence of Adult Attachment on Symptom Reporting: Testing a Mediational Model in a Sample of the General Population." *Psychology and Health* 21(3):351–366.

Armitage, Christopher J., Mark Conner, Justin Loach, and David Willetts. 1999. "Different Perceptions of Control: Applying an Extended Theory of Planned Behavior to Legal and Illegal Drug Use." *Basic & Applied Social Psychology* 21(4):301–316.

Arnett, J. 1991. "Heavy Metal Music and Reckless Behavior among Adolescents." *Journal of Youth and Adolescence*, 20(6):573–592.

Arseth, Annie K., Jane Kroger, Monica Martinussen, and Guro Bakken. 2009. "Intimacy Status, Attachment, Separation-Individuation Patterns, and Identity Status in Female University Students." *Journal of Social & Personal Relationships* 26(5):697–712.

Arthur, James. 2008. "Traditional Approaches to Character Education in Britain and America." pp. 80–98 in *Handbook of Moral and Character Education*, edited by Larry P. Nucci and Darcia Narvaez. New York: Routledge.

Ashe, D. D., and L. E. McCutcheon. 2001. Shyness, Loneliness, and Attitude toward Celebrities." *Current Research in Social Psychology* 6(9):124–133.

Aslan, Sevda, 2015. "The Prediction of Separation-Individuation through Internal-External Locus of Control in Turkish Late Adolescents." *Journal of Psychological & Educational Research* 23(2):73–89.

Atkin, C., and M. Block. 1983. "Effectiveness of Celebrity Endorsers." *Journal of Advanced Research* 23(1):57–61.

Attar-Schwartz, Shalhevet, Jo-Pei Tan, and Ann Buchanan. 2009. "Adolescents' Perspectives on Relationships with Grandparents: The Contribution of Adolescent Grandparent and Parent-grandparent Relationship Variables." *Children & Youth Service Review* 31:1057–1066.

Augustyn, M. B., and J. M. McGloin. 2013. "The Risk of Informal Socializing with Peers: Considering Gender Differences Across Predatory Delinquency and Substance Use." *Justice Quarterly* 30(1):117–143.

Austin, Erica Weintraub, Rebecca Van de Vord, Bruce E. Pinkleton, and Evan Epstein. 2008. "Celebrity Endorsements and Their Potential to Motivate Young Voters." *Mass Communication & Society* 11:420–436.

Awang, Mohd Mahzan, Abdul Razaq Ahmad, Nora'asikin Abu Bakar, Sayuti Abd Ghani, Asyraf Nadia Mohd Yunus, et al. 2013. "Students' Attitudes and Their Academic Performance in Nationhood Education." *International Education Studies* 6(11):21–28.

Axinn, William, Jennifer S. Barber, and Arland Thornton. 1999. "Values and Beliefs as Determinants of Outcomes in Children's Lives." pp. 118–127 in *Transitions to Adulthood in a Changing Economy: No Work, No Family, No Future?*, edited by Alan Booth, Ann C. Crouter, and Michael J. Shanahan. Westport, CT: Praeger.

Azfredrick, Ezinwanne Christiana. 2015. "Use of Counselling Services by School-Attending Adolescent Girls in Nigeria." *Journal of Child & Adolescent Mental Health* 27(1):1–10.

Baartman, Liesbeth, and Lotte Ruijs. 2011. "Comparing Students' Perceived and Actual Competence in Higher Vocational Education." *Assessment & Evaluation in Higher Education* 36(4):385–398.

Baer, Judith. 2002. "Is Family Cohesion a Risk or Protection Factor during Adolescent Development?" *Journal of Marriage & Family* 64(3):668–675.

Bagwell, Catherine L., and Michelle E. Schmidt. 2011. *Friendships in Childhood & Adolescence*. New York: Guilford.

Balswick, Jack, and Bron Ingoldsby. 1982. "Heroes and Heroines among American Adolescents." *Sex Roles* 8(3):243–249.

Bandura, A. 1977. "Self-efficacy: Toward a Unifying Theory of Behavioral Change." *Psychological Review* 84(2):191.

Bandura, A. 1986. "The Explanatory and Predictive Scope of Self-Efficacy Theory." *Journal of Social and Clinical Psychology* 4(3):359.

Bandura, A. 1993. "Perceived Self-efficacy in Cognitive Development and Functioning." *Educational Psychologist* 28(2):117–148.

Bandura, A. 1997. *Self-efficacy: The Exercise of Control*. Macmillan.

Barrett, Martyn. 2007. *Children's Knowledge, Beliefs and Feelings about Nations and National Groups*. Hove, UK: Psychology Press.

Barry, Carolyn McNamara, and Allan Wigfield. 2002. "Social Perceptions of Friendship-making Ability and Perceptions of Friends' Deviant Behavior: Childhood to Adolescence." *Journal of Early Adolescence* 22(2):143–172.

Bartholomew, K. 1990. "Avoidance of Intimacy: An Attachment Perspective." *Journal of Social and Personal Relationships* 7(2):147–178.

Bartholomew, K., and L. M. Horowitz. 1991. "Attachment Styles among Young Adults: A Test of a Four-category Model." *Journal of Personality and Social Psychology* 61(2):226.

Batey, M., T. Chamorro-Premuzic, and A. Furnham. 2009. "Intelligence and Personality as Predictors of Divergent Thinking: The Role of General, Fluid and Crystallised Intelligence." *Thinking Skills and Creativity* 4(1):60–69.

Batson, C. D., and P. Scheonrade. 1991a. "Measuring Religion as Quest: 1) Validity Concerns." *Journal for the Scientific Study of Religion* 30:416–429.

Batson, C. D., and P. Scheonrade. 1991b. "Measuring Religion as Quest: 2) Reliability Concerns." *Journal for the Scientific Study of Religion* 30:430–447.

Batson, C. D., P. Scheonrade, and W. L. Ventis. 1993. *Religion and the Individual: A Social Psychological Perspective*. London: Oxford University Press.

Bauman, Zygmunt. 2005. *Work, Consumerism and the New Poor*. Maidenhead, UK: Open University Press.

Bauminger, Nirit, Ricky Finzi-Dottan, Sagit Chason, and Dov Har-Even. 2008. "Intimacy in Adolescent Friendship: The Roles of Attachment, Coherence, and Self-Disclosure." *Journal of Social & Personal Relationships* 25(3):409–428.

Beck, R. 2006. "God as a Secure Base: Attachment to God and Theological Exploration." *Journal of Psychology and Theology* 34(2):125–132.

Beck, R., and A. McDonald. 2004. "Attachment to God: The Attachment to God Inventory, Tests of Working Model Correspondence, and an Exploration of Faith Group Differences." *Journal of Psychology and Theology* 32(2):92–103.

Becker, Kolf, and Anna Etta Hecken. 2009. "Higher Education or Vocational Training? An Empirical Test of the Rational Action Model of Educational Choices Suggested by Breen and Goldthorpe and Esser." *Acta Sociologica* 52(1):25–45.

Bellair, Paul E., and Vincent J. Roscigno. 2000. "Local Labor-Market Opportunity and Adolescent Delinquency." *Social Forces* 78(4):1509–1538.

Benda, Brent B. 2002. "A Test of Three Competing Theoretical Models of Delinquency Using Structural Equation Modeling." *Journal of Social Service Research* 29(2):55–91.

Benda, Brent B., and Robert Flynn Corwyn. 2002. "The Effect of Abuse in Childhood and in Adolescence on Violence among Adolescents." *Youth & Society* 33(2):339–365.

Bendicksen, Harold K. 2013. *The Transformational Self-attachment and the End of the Adolescent Phase*. London: Karnac.

Bensley, D. Alan, and Cheryl Haynes. 1995. "The Acquisition of General Purpose Strategic Knowledge for Argumentation." *Teaching of Psychology* 22(1):41–45.

Benson, Janel E. 2007. "Make New Friends but Keep the Old: Peers and the Transition to College." *Advances in Life Course Research* 12:309–334.

Benson, Peter L., Peter C. Scales, and Amy K. Syvertsen. 2011. "The Contribution of the Developmental Assets Framework to Positive Youth Development Theory and Practice." *Advances in Child Development & Behavior* 197–230.

Berger, C. R. 1986. "Uncertain Outcome Values in Predicted Relationships Uncertainty Reduction Theory Then and Now." *Human Communication Research* 13(1):34–38.

Berger, C. R., and R. J. Calabrese. 1975. "Some Explorations in Initial Interaction and Beyond: Towards a Development Theory of Interpersonal Communication." *Human Communication Research* 1:99–112.

Berger, Jonah, and Chip Heath. 2008. "Who Drives Divergence? Identity Signaling, Outgroup Dissimilarity, and the Abandonment of Cultural Tastes." *Journal of Personality & Social Psychology* 95(3):593–607.

Berger, S. M. 1977. "Social Comparison, Modeling, and Perservance." pp. 209–234 in *Social Comparison Processes: Theoretical and Empirical Perspectives*, edited by J. M. Suls and R. L. Miller. Washington DC: Hemisphere.

Berkowitz, Marvin W., Victor A. Battistich, and Melinda C. Bier. 2008. "What Works in Character Education: What Is Known and What Needs to Be Known." pp. 414–431 in *Handbook of Moral and Character Education*, edited by Larry P. Nucci and Darcia Narvaez. New York: Routledge.

Bernardon, Stephanie, Kimberley A. Babb, Julie Hakim-Larson, Marcia Gragg. 2011. "Loneliness, Attachment, and the Perception and Use of Social Support in University Students." *Canadian Journal of Behavioural Science* 43(1):40–51.

Bhanot, Ruchi T., and Jasna Jovanovic. 2009. "The Link between Parent Behaviors and Boys' and Girls' Science Achievement Beliefs." *Applied Developmental Science* 13(1):42–59.

Bidmon, Sonja. 2017. "How Does Attachment Style Influence the Brand Attachment: Brand Trust and Brand Loyalty Chain in Adolescents?" *International Journal of Advertising* 36(1):164–189.

Bidwell, Charles E., Stephen Plank, and Chandra Muller. 1996. "Peer Social Networks and Adolescent Career Development." pp. 107–131 in *Generating Social Stratification: Toward a New Research Agenda*, edited by Alan C. Kerckhoff. Boulder, CO: Westview.

Bjarnason, Thoroddur. 2009. "Anomie among European Adolescents: Conceptual and Empirical Clarification of a Multilevel Sociological Concept." *Sociological Forum* 24(1):135–161.

Bleich, Susan, Dolf Zillmann, and James Weaver. 1991. "Enjoyment and Consumption of Defiant Rock Music as a Function of Adolescent Rebelliousness." *Journal of Broadcasting & Electronic Media* 35:351–366.

Blinde, Elaine M. 1995. "Teaching Sociology of Sport: An Active Learning Approach." *Teaching Sociology* 23(3):264–268.

Blos, P. 1967. "The Second Individuation Process of Adolescence." *The Psychoanalytic Study of the Child* 22(1):162–186.

Bodovski, Katerina. 2010. "Parental Practices and Educational Achievement: Social Class, Race, and Habitus." *British Journal of Sociology of Education* 31(2):139–156.

Bokhorst, Caroline L., Sindy R. Sumter, and P. Michael Westenberg. 2009. "Social Support from Parents, Friends, Classmates, and Teachers in Children and Adolescents Aged 9 to 18 Years: Who Is Perceived as Most Supportive?" *Social Development* 19(2):417–426.

Bonds-Raacke, Jennifer M., Erica S. Bearden, Noelle J. Carriere, Ellen M. Anderson, and Sandra D. Nicks. 2001. "Engaging Distortions: Are We Idealizing Marriage?" *Journal of Psychology* 135(2):179–184.

Boon, Susan D., and Christine D. Lomore. 2001. "Admirer-celebrity Relationships among Young Adults: Explaining Perceptions of Celebrity Influence on Identity." *Human Communication Research* 27(3):432–465.

Boone, Liesbet. 2013. "Are Attachment Styles Differentially Related to Interpersonal Perfectionism and Binge Eating Symptoms?" *Personality & Individual Differences* 54(8):931–935.

Bouchard, Martin, Wei Wang, and Eric Beauregard. 2012. "Social Capital, Opportunity, and School-Based Victimization." *Violence & Victims* 27(5):656–673.

Bourdieu, Pierre. 1979. *Distinction: A Social Critique of the Judgment of Taste.* London: Routledge.

Bowers, David M., Daniel A. Rosch, and Jill R. Collier. 2016. "Examining the Relationship between Role Models and Leadership Growth during the Transition to Adulthood." *Journal of Adolescent Research* 31(1):96–118.

Bowlby, J. 1969. *Attachment: Attachment and Loss,* Vol. 1. New York: Basic Books, Chapter 5.

Bowlby, J. 1973. *Attachment and Loss.* Vol. 2. New York: Basic Books.

Bowman, W. D. 1998. *Philosophical Perspectives on Music.* New York: Oxford University Press.

Bradley, Robert H., Bettye M. Caldwell, and Stephen L. Rock. 1988. "Home Environment and School Performance: A Ten-Year Follow-up and Examination of Three Models of Environmental Action." *Child Development* 59:852–867.

Bradley, Robert H., Robert F. Corwyn, Bettye M. Caldwell, Leanne Whiteside-Mansell, Gail A. Wasserman, and Iris T. Mink. 2000. "Measuring the Home Environments of Children in Early Adolescence." *Journal of Research in Adolescence* 10(3):247–288.

Branner, Julia, and Ann Nilsen. 2005. "Individualisation, Choice and Structure: A Discussion of Current Trends on Sociological Analysis." *Sociological Review* 35:412–428.

Braunstein-Bercovitz, Hedva, Benny A. Benjamin, Shiri Asor, and Maya Lev. 2012. "Insecure Attachment and Career Indecision: Mediating Effects of Anxiety and Pessimism." *Journal of Vocational Behavior* 81:236–244.

Brendgen, Mara, Frank Vitaro, and William M. Bukowski. 2000. "Deviant Friends and Early Adolescents' Emotional and Behavioral Adjustment." *Journal of Research on Adolescence* 10(2):173–189.

Brennan, K. A., and J. K. Bosson. 1998. "Attachment-style Differences in Attitudes toward and Reactions to Feedback from Romantic Partners: An Exploration of the Relational Bases of Self-esteem." *Personality and Social Psychology Bulletin* 24(7):699–714.

Brennan, K. A., and K. A. Morris. 1997. "Attachment Styles, Self-esteem, and Patterns of Seeking Feedback from Romantic Partners." *Personality and Social Psychology Bulletin* 23(1):23–31.

Brennan, Lauretta M., and Daneil S. Shaw. 2015. "Prenatal and Early Childhood Prevention of Antisocial Behavior." pp. 351–369 in *The Handbook Juvenile Delinquency and Juvenile Justice*, edited by Marvin D. Krohn and Jodi Lane. Chichester, UK: Wiley.

Brensilver, Matthew, Sonya Negriff, Ferol E. Mennen, and Penelope K. Trickett. 2011. "Longitudinal Relations between Depressive Symptoms and Externalizing Behavior in Adolescence: Moderating Effects of Maltreatment Experience and Gender." *Journal of Clinical Child & Adolescent Psychology* 40(4):607–617.

Bringle, R. G., and G. J. Bagby. 1992. "Self-esteem and Perceived Quality of Romantic and Family Relationships in Young Adults." *Journal of Research in Personality* 26(4):340–356.

Broh, Beckett A. 2002. "Linking Extracurricular Programming to Academic Achievement: Who Benefits and Why?" *Sociology of Education* 75(1):69–91.

Broidy, Lisa M. 2001. "A Test of General Strain Theory." *Criminology* 39(1):9–35.

Bronuer, Stephen Eric. 2002. "Sketching the Lineage: The Critical Method and the Idealist Tradition." *New Political Science* 24(2):265–292.

Brookfield, Stephen D. 1987. *Developing Critical Thinkers: Challenging Adults to Explore Alternative Ways of Thinking and Acting*. Milton Keynes, UK: Open University Press.

Brouwers, Symen A., Ramesh C. Mishra, and Fons J.R. Van de Vijver. 2006. "Schooling and Everyday Cognitive Development among Kharwar Children in India: A Natural Experiment." *International Journal of Behavioral Development* 30(6):559–567.

Brown, Olivia K. and Douglas K. Symons. 2016. "My Pet Has Passed: Relations of Adult Attachment Styles and Current Feelings of Grief and Trauma after the Event." *Death Studies* 40(4):247–255.

Browne, M. Neil. 2000. "Distinguishing Features of Critical Thinking Classrooms." *Teaching in Higher Education* 5(3):301–309.

Buist, Kristen L., Maja Dekovic, Wim H. Meeus, and Marcel A. G. van Aken. 2004. "Attachment in Adolescence: A Social Relations Model Analysis." *Journal of Adolescent Research* 19(6):826–850.

Bunge, Mario. 1996. *Finding Philosophy in Social Science*. New Haven, CT: Yale University Press.

Burger, Kaspar, and Robin Samuel. 2017. "The Role of Perceived Stress and Self-Efficacy in Young People's Life Satisfaction: A Longitudinal Study." *Journal of Youth & Adolescence* 46(1):78–90.

Burgess, Simon, Carol Propper, and Karen Gardiner. 2006. "School, Family and County Effects on Adolescents' Later Life Chances." *Journal of Family & Economic Issues* 27(2):155–184.

Busch, Fredric N. 2009. "Anger and Depression." *Advances in Psychiatric Treatment* 15(4):271–278.

Bush, Alan J., Craig A. Martin, and Victoria D. Bush. 2005. "Sports Celebrity Influence on the Behavioral Intentions of Generation Y." *Journal of Advertising Research* 45:108–118.

Bush, Kevin, Gary W. Peterson, Jose A. Cobas, and Andrew J. Supple. 2002. "Adolescents' Perceptions of Parental Behaviors as Predictors of Adolescent Self-esteem in Mainland China." *Sociological Inquiry* 72(4):503–526.

Buxton, David. [1983] 1990. "Rock Music, the Star System, and the Rise of Consumerism." pp. 427–440 in *On Record: Rock, Pop, and the Written Word*, edited by Simon Frith and Andrew Goodwin. London: Routledge.

Bylsma, W. H., C. Cozzarelli, and N. Sumer. 1997. "Relation between Adult Attachment Styles and Global Self-esteem." *Basic and Applied Social Psychology* 19(1):1–16.

Bynner, John, and Samantha Parsons. 2002. "Social Exclusion and the Transition from School to Work: The Case of Young People Not in Education, Employment, or Training (NEET)." *Journal of Vocational Behavior* 60:289–309.

Callas, Peter W., Brian S. Flynn, and John K. Worden. 2004. "Potentially Modifiable Psychosocial Factors Associated with Alcohol Use during Early Adolescence." *Addictive Behaviors* 29:1503–1515.

Calvert, Sandra L., Katherine J. Murray, and Emily E. Conger. 2004. "Heroic DVD Portrayals: What US and Taiwanese Adolescents Admire and Understand." *Applied Developmental Psychology* 25:699–716.

Calvert, Sandra L., Tracy A. Kondla, Karen A. Ertel, and Douglas S. Meisel. 2001. "Young Adults' Perceptions and Memories of a Televised Woman Hero." *Sex Roles* 45(1–2):31–52.

Cambon, Laurent, Vincent Yzerbyt, and Sonya Yakimova. 2015. "Compensation in Intergroup Relations: An Investigation of Its Structural and Strategic Foundations." *British Journal of Social Psychology* 54(1):140–158.

Campbell, Heather E. 2004. "Prices, Devices, People, or Rules: The Relative Effectiveness of Policy Instruments in Water Conservation." *Review of Policy Research* 21(5):637–662.

Campbell, Mary E., and Jennifer Eggerling-Boeck. 2006. "What about the Children? The Psychological and Social Well-being of Multiracial Adolescents." *Sociological Quarterly* 47:147–173.

Cao, Zidan, and Shunan Wang. 1993. *Summary of Studies of Causes of Crime in China.* Qinhuangdao, China: China Political Legal University.

Caplan, Leslie J., and Carmi Schooler. 2007. "Socioeconomic Status and Financial Coping Strategies: The Mediating Role of Perceived Control." *Social Psychology Quarterly* 70(1):43–58.

Carlo, Gustavo, Meredith McGinley, Rachel C. Hayes, and Miriam M. Martinez. 2012. "Empathy as a Mediator of the Relations between Parent and Peer Attachment and Prosocial and Physically Aggressive Behaviors in Mexican American College Students." *Journal of Social & Personal Relationships* 29(3):337–357.

Carvajal, Scott C., Carrie Hanson, Roberta A. Downing, Karin K. Coyle, and Linda L. Pederson. 2004. "Theory-based Determinants of Youth Smoking: A Multiple Influence Approach." *Journal of Applied Social Psychology* 34(1):59–84.

Catalano, Richard F., James J. Mazza, Tracy W. Harachi, Robert D. Abbott, Kevin P. Haggerty, and Charles B. Fleming. 2003. "Raising Healthy Children through Enhancing Social Development in Elementary School: Results after 1.5 Years." *Journal of School Psychology* 41:143–164.

Cattarello, Anne M. 2000. "Community-level Influences in Individuals' Social Bonds, Peer Associations, and Delinquency: A Multilevel Analysis." *Justice Quarterly* 17(1):35–60.

Cavanagh, Shannon E. 2007. "The Social Construction of Romantic Relationships in Adolescence: Examining the Role of Peer Networks, Gender, and Race." *Sociological Inquiry* 77(4):572–600.

Cavanagh, Shannon E. 2011. "Early Puberty Timing and the Union Formation Behaviors of Young Women." *Social Forces* 89(4):1217–1238.

Chan, David W. 2008. "Emotional Intelligence, Self-efficacy, and Coping among Chinese Prospective and In-service Teachers in Hong Kong." *Educational Psychology* 28(4):391–408.

Chan, Elaine. 2001. "Defining Fellow Compatriots 'Others': National Identity in Hong Kong." *Government and Opposition* 35(4):499–519.

Chan, W. T., C. K. Cheung, T. Y. Lee, K. K. Leung, and S. C. Liu. 1998. *Moral Values of Youth in Hong Kong*. Hong Kong: Department of Applied Social Studies, City University of Hong Kong.

Chang, Tzu-Fen, Eun-Jin Han, Jin-Suk Lee, and Desiree B. Qin. 2015. "Korean American Adolescent Ethnic-Identity Pride and Psychological Adjustment: Moderating Effects of Parental Support and School Environment." *Asian American Journal of Psychology* 6(2):190–199.

Chappelle, W. L., M. P. L. Novy, C. T. W. Sowin, and W. T. Thompson. 2010. "NEO PI-R Normative Personality Data that Distinguish US Air Force Female Pilots." *Military Psychology* 22(2):158.

Charles, Camille Z., Gniesha, Dinwiddie, and Douglas S. Massey. 2004. "The Continuing Consequences of Segregation: Family Stress and College Academic Performance." *Social Science Quarterly* 85(5):1353–1373.

Chen, Zeng-yin, Sanford M. Dornbusch, and Ruth X. Liu. 2007. "Direct and Indirect Patways between Parental Constructive: Behavior and Adolescent Affiliation with Achievement-oriented Peers." *Journal of Child & Family Studies* 16:837–858.

Cheng, E., R. Stebbins, and J. Packer. 2017. "Serious Leisure among Older Gardeners in Australia." *Leisure Studies* 36(4):505–518.

Cheng, F. 2017. *Identificatory Idol Worship and the Self: A Multi-faceted Study of Their Relationship*. Undergraduate Thesis, City University of Hong Kong.

Cheng, S. 1997. "Psychological Determinants of Idolatry in Adolescents." *Adolescence* 32(127):687–692.

Cheung, C. K., and X. D. Yue. 1999. "Idol Worshipping for Vain Glory, Illusory Romance or Intellectual Learning: A Study in Nanjing and Hong Kong." *International Journal of Adolescence and Youth* 7:20–28.

Cheung, C. K., and X. D. Yue. 2000. "Idol Worshipping for Vain Glory, Illusory Romance or Intellectual Learning: A Study in Nanjing and Hong Kong." *International Journal of Adolescence and Youth* 8(4):299–317.

Cheung, C. K., and X. D. Yue. 2003a. "Adolescent Modeling after Luminary and Star Idols and Development of Self-Efficacy." *International Journal of Adolescence and Youth*, 11(3):251–267.

Cheung, C. K., and X. D. Yue. 2003b. "Identity Achievement and Idol Worship among Teenagers in Hong Kong." *International Journal of Adolescence and Youth* 11(1):1–26.

Cheung, C. K., and X. D. Yue. 2004. Adolescent Modeling after Luminary and Star Idols and Development of Self-Efficacy. *International Journal of Adolescence and Youth* 11:251–267.

Cheung, C. K., and X. D. Yue. 2011. "Pentangular Dimensions of Chinese Adolescents' Idol Worship." *International Journal of Adolescence and Youth* 16:225–244.

Cheung, C. K., and X. D. Yue. 2012. "Idol Worship as Compensation for Parental Absence." *International Journal of Adolescence and Youth* 17(1):35–46.

Cheung, C. K., and X. D. Yue. 2018. "Idols as Sunshine or Road Signs: Comparing Absorption-Addiction Idolatry with Identification-Emulation Idolatry." *Psychological Reports*, 0033294118758903.

Cheung, Cecilia Sin-Sze, and Eva M. Pomerantz. 2011. "Parents' Involvement in Children's Learning in the United States and China: Applications for Children's Academic and Emotional Adjustment." *Child Development* 82(3):332–350.

Cheung, G. W., and R. B. Rensvold. 2002. "Evaluating Goodness-of-Fit Indexes for Testing Measurement Invariance." *Structural Equation Modeling* 9:233–255.

Cheung, Kelvin Chi-Kin. 2015. "Child Poverty in Hong Kong Single-Parent Families." *Child Indicators Research* 8(3):517–536.

Ching, H. C. 2008. *A Study of the Relationship of Idol Worship, Ego Identity and Self-efficacy amongst 184 Adolescents in Hong Kong.* Undergraduate Thesis, City University of Hong Kong.

Chiou, Jyh-shen, Chien-yi Huang, and Min-chieh Chuang. 2005. "Antecedents of Taiwanese Adolescents' Purchase Intention toward the Merchandise of a Celebrity: The Moderating Effect of Celebrity Adoration." *Journal of Social Psychology* 45(3):317–332.

Choo, Hyekyung, and Daniel Shek. 2013. "Quality of Parent-child Relationship, Family Conflict, Peer Pressure, and Drinking Behaviors of Adolescents in an Asian Context: The Case of Singapore." *Social Indicators Research* 110:1141–1159.

Chou, Kee-Lee. 2000. "Intimacy and Psychosocial Adjustment in Hong Kong Chinese Adolescents." *Journal of Genetic Psychology* 161(2):141–151.

Chow, Chong Man, Ellen Hart, Lillian Ellis, and Cin Cin Tan. 2017. "Interdependence of Attachment Styles and Relationship Quality in Parent-Adolescent Dyads." *Journal of Adolescence* 61:77–86.

Christopher, F. Scott, Franklin O. Poulsen, and Sarah J. McKenney. 2016. "Early Adolescents and Going out: The Emergence of Romantic Relationship Roles." *Journal of Social & Personal Relationships* 33(6):814–834.

Chuang, Yao-Chia. 2005. "Effects of Interaction Pattern in Family Harmony and Well-being: Test of Interpersonal Theory, Relational Models Theory, and Confucian Ethics." *Asian Journal of Social Psychology* 8:272–291.

Chui, Wing Hong, and Heng Choon Oliver Chan. 2012. "An Empirical Investigation of Social Bonds and Juvenile Delinquency in Hong Kong." *Child & Youth Care Forum* 41:371–386.

Chui, Wing Hong, and Heng Choon (Oliver) Chan. 2016. "The Gendered Analysis of Self-Control on Theft and Violent Delinquency: An Examination of Hong Kong Adolescent Population." *Crime & Delinquency* 62(12):1648–1677.

Chui, Wing Hong, and Matthew Y. H. Wong. 2017. "Avoiding Disappointment or Fulfilling Expectation: A Study of Gender, Academic Achievement, and Family Functioning among Hong Kong Adolescents." *Journal of Child & Family Studies* 26(1):48–56.

Cikrikci, Özkan, and Hatice Odaci. 2016. "The Determinants of Life Satisfaction among Adolescents: The Role of Metacognitive Awareness and Self-Efficacy." *Social Indicators Research* 125(3):977–990.

Clark, Paul. 2012. *Youth Culture in China: From Red Guards to Netizens.* New York: Cambridge University Press.

Cohen, Geoffrey L., and Mitchell J. Prinstein. 2006. "Peer Contagion of Aggression and Health Risk Behavior among Adolescent Males: An Experimental Investigation of Effects on Public Conduct and Private Attitudes." *Child Development* 77(4):967–983.

Cohen, Jonathan. 2004. "Parasocial Break-up from Favorite Television Characters: The Role of Attachment Styles and Relationship Intensity." *Journal of Social & Personal Relationships* 21(2):187–202.

Cole, Tim, and Laura Leets. 1999. "Attachment Styles and Intimate Television Viewing: Insecurely Forming Relationships in a Parasocial Way." *Journal of Social & Personal Relationships* 16(4):495–511.

Collins, N. L. 2002. "Psychosocial Vulnerability from Adolescence to Adulthood: A Prospective Study of Attachment Style Differences in Relationship Functioning and Partner Choice." *Journal of Personality* 70(6):965–1008.

Collins, N. L., and S. J. Read. 1990. "Adult Attachment, Working Models, and Relationship Quality in Dating Couples." *Journal of Personality and Social Psychology* 58(4):644.

Collins, Nancy L., and Brooke C. Feeney. 2000. "A Safe Haven: An Attachment Theory Perspective on Support Seeking and Caregiving in Intimate Relationships." *Journal of Personality & Social Psychology* 78(6):1053–1073.

Collins, W. Andrew, and Manfred van Dulmen. 2006. "The Significance of Middle Childhood Peer Competence for Work and Relationships in Early Adulthood." pp. 23–40 in *Developmental Contexts in Middle Childhood: Bridges to Adolescence and Adulthood*, edited by Aletha C. Huston and Marika N. Ripke. Cambridge, UK: Cambridge University Press.

Conger, Rand D., and Katherine J. Conger. 2002. "Resilience in Midwestern Families: Selected Findings from the First Decade of a Prospective, Longitudinal Study." *Journal of Marriage & Family* 64(2):361–373.

Connell, Arin M., and Thomas J. Dishion. 2006. "The Contribution of Peers to Monthly Variation in Adolescent Depressed Mood: A Short-term Longitudinal Study with Time-varying Predictors." *Development & Psychopathology* 18:139–154.

Cornell, Dewey G., Peter J. Lovegrove, Michael W. Baly. 2014. "Invalid Survey Response Patterns among Middle School Students." *Psychological Assessment* 26(1):277–287.

Costello, Barbara J., and Paul R. Vowell. 1999. "Testing Control Theory and Differential Association: A Reanalysis of the Richmond Youth Project Data." *Criminology* 37(4):815–842.

Cote, James. 2014. *Youth Studies: Fundamental Issues and Debates.* Houndmills, UK: Palgrave.

Cotterell, John L. 1992. "School Size as a Factor in Adolescents' Adjustment to the Transition to Secondary School." *Journal of Early Adolescence* 12(1):28–45.

Cotterell, John. 2007. *Social Networks in Youth and Adolescence*, 2nd ed. London: Routledge.

Cradock, Angie L., Ichiro Kawachi, Graham A. Colditz, Steven L. Gortmaker, and Stephen L. Buka. 2009. "Neighborhood Social Cohesion and Youth Participation in Physical Activity in Chicago." *Social Science & Medicine* 68:427–435.

Creed, Peter A., and Wendy Patton. 2003. "Predicting Two Components of Career Maturity in School-based Adolescents." *Journal of Career Development* 29(4):277–290.

Croghan, Rosaleen, Christine Griffin, Janine Hunter, and Ann Phoenix. 2006. "Single Failure: Consumption, Identity and Social Exclusion." *Journal of Youth Studies* 9(4):463–478.

Crompton, Rosemary. 1996. "Consumption and Class Analysis." pp. 113–132 in *Consumption Matters: The Production and Experience of Consumption*, edited by Stephen Edgell, Kevin Hetherington, and Alan Warde. Oxford, UK: Blackwell.

Crosnoe, Robert, and Glen A. Elder, Jr. 2004. "Family Dynamics, Supportive Relationships, and Educational Resilience during Adolescence." *Journal of Family Issues* 25(5):574–602.

Crosnoe, Robert, Rashmita S. Mistry, and Glen H. Elder, Jr. 2002. "Economic Disadvantage, Family Dynamics, and Adolescent Enrollment in Higher Education." *Journal of Marriage & Family* 64(3):690–702.

Cruce, Ty M., and John V. Moore, III. 2007. "First-year Students' Plans to Volunteer: An Examination of the Prediction of Community Service Participation." *Journal of College Student Development* 48(6):655–673.

Crystal, David S., and Matthew DeBell. 2002. "Sources of Civic Orientation among American Youth: Trust, Religious Valuation, and Attributions of Responsibility." *Political Psychology* 23(1):113–132.

Csikai, Ellen L., and Cindy Rosensky. 1997. "Social Work Idealism and Students' Perceived Reasons for Entering Social Work." *Journal of Social Work Education* 33(3):529–538.

Cui, Naixue, Jia Xue, Cynthia A. Connolly, and Jianghong Li. 2016. "Does the Gender of Parent or Child Matter in Child Maltreatment in China?" *Child Abuse & Neglect* 54:1–9.

Cusick, Linda. 2002. "Youth Prostitution: A Literature Review." *Child Abuse Review* 11:230–251.

Dacey, John S., and Kathleen H. Lennon. 1998. *Understanding Creativity: The Interplay of Biological, Psychological, and Social Factors.* San Francisco, CA: Jossey-Bass.

Danes, Sharon M., Michael C. Rodriguez, and Katherine E. Brewton. 2013. "Learning Context When Studying Financial Planning in High Schools: Nesting of Student, Teacher, and Classroom Characteristics." *Journal of Financial Counseling & Planning* 24(2):20–36.

Davidson, W. P. 1983. "The Third-Person Effect in Communication." *Public Opinion Quarterly* 47:1–15.

De Backer, Charlotte J. S. 2012. "Blinded by the Starlight: An Evolutionary Framework for Studying Celebrity Culture and Fandom." *Review of General Psychology* 16(2):144–151.

De Backer, Charlotte J. S., Mark Nelissen, Patrick Vyncke, Johan Braeckman, and Francis T. McAndrew. 2007. "Celebrities: From Teachers to Friends: A Test of Two Hypotheses on the Adaptiveness of Celebrity Gossip." *Human Nature* 18(4):334–354.

De Bruyn, Eddy H., and Dymphna C. van den Boom. 2005. "Interpersonal Behavior, Peer Popularity, and Self-esteem in Early Adolescence." *Social Development* 14(4):555–573.

De Bruyn, Eddy H., Maia Dekovic, G. Wim Meijnen. 2003. "Parenting, Goal Orientations, Classroom Behavior, and School Success in Early Adolescence." *Applied Developmental Psychology* 24:393–412.

de Jong, Marjolein L. 1992. "Attachment, Individuation, and Risk of Suicide in Late Adolescence." *Journal of Youth and Adolescence* 21(3):357–373.

Diener, Marissa L., M. Angela Nievar, and Cheryl Wright. 2003. "Attachment Security among Mothers and Their Young Children Living in Poverty: Associations with Maternal Child, and Contextual Characteristics." *Merrill-Palmer Quarterly* 49(2):154–182.

DiRenzo, Marco S., Christy H. Weer, and Frank Linnehan. 2013. "Protégé Career Aspirations: The Influence of Formal E-Mentor Networks and Family-Based Role Models." *Journal of Vocational Behavior* 83(1):41–50.

DiTommaso, E., C. Brannen-McNulty, L. Ross, and M. Burgess. 2003. "Attachment Styles, Social Skills and Loneliness in Young Adults." *Personality and Individual Differences* 35(2):303–312.

Donay, Lloyd D., and Noreen E. Lephardt. 1993. "Developing Critical Thinking Skills in Accounting Students." *Journal of Education for Business* 68(5):297–300.

Dorahy, Martin J., Christopher Alan Lewis, Robert G. Millar, and Travis L. Gee. 2003. "Predictors of Nonpathological Dissociation in Northern Ireland: The Effects of Trauma and Exposure to Political Violence." *Journal of Traumatic Stress* 16(6):611–615.

Dorius, Guy L., and Tim B. Heaton. 1993. "Adolescent Life Events and Their Association with the Onset of Sexual Intercourse." *Youth & Society* 25(1):3–35.

Downing, Haley M., and Margaret M. Nauta. 2010. "Separation-Individuation, Exploration, and Identity Diffusion as Mediators of the Relationship between Attachment and Career Indecision." *Journal of Career Development* 36(3):207–227.

Driscoll, Catherine. 1999. "Girl Culture, Revenge, and Global Capitalism: Cybergirls, Riot Grrls, Spice Girls." *Australian Feminist Studies* 14(29):173–194.

Dufur, Mikaela J., Toby L. Parcel, and Benjamin A. McKune. 2013. "Does Capital at Home Matter More Than Capital at School? The Case of Adolescent Alcohol and Marijuana Use." *Journal of Drug Issues* 43(1):85–102.

Dumais, Susan A. 2006. "Elementary School Students' Extracurricular Activities: The Effect of Participation on Achievement and Teachers' Evaluations." *Sociological Spectrum* 26:117–147.

Dunkel, Curtis S., Aaron W. Lukaszewski, and Kristine Chua. 2016. "The Relationships between Sex, Life History Strategy, and Adult Romantic Attachment Style." *Personality & Individual Differences* 98:176–178.

Dunn, Jacquie, Vivienne Lewis, and Sally Patrick. 2010. "The Idealization of Thin Figures and Appearance Concerns in Middle School Children." *Journal of Applied Biobehavioral Research* 15(3):134–143.

Dupree, Davido, Margaret Beale Spencer, and Suzanne Fegley. 2007. "Perceived Social Inequity and Responses to Conflict among Diverse Youth of Color: The Effects of Social and Physical Context on Youth Behavior and Attitudes." pp. 111–131 *in Approaches to Positive Youth Development*, edited by Rainer K. Silbereisen and Richard M. Lerner. Thousand Oaks, CA: Sage.

Durlak, Joseph A., Rebecca D. Taylor, Kei Kawashima, Molly K. Pachlan, Emily P. DuPre, Christine I. Celio, Sasha R. Berger, Allison B. Dymnicki, and Peter P. Weissberg. 2007. "Effects of Positive Youth Development Programs on School, Family, and Community Systems." *American Journal of Community Psychology* 39:269–286.

Earl, Jennifer, and Katrina Kimport. 2009. "Movement Societies and Digital Protest: Fan Activism and Other Nonpolitical Protest Online." *Sociological Theory* 27(3):220–243.

East, Patricia L. 2009. "Adolescents' Relationships with Siblings." pp. 43–73 in *Handbook of Adolescent Psychology, Vol.2: Contextual Influences and Adolescent Development*, edited by Richard M. Lerner and Laurence Steinberg. Hoboken, NJ: Wiley.

Eberly, Mary B., and Raymond Montemayor. 1998. "Doing Good Deeds: An Examination of Adolescent Prosocial Behavior in the Context of Parent-adolescent Relationships." *Journal of Adolescent Research* 13(4):403–432.

Eccles, Jacquelynne. 1985. "Sex Differences in Achievement Pattern." pp. 97–132 in *Psychology and Gender, Nebraska Symposium on Motivation*, 1984, edited by Theo B. Sonderegger. Lincoln, NB: University of Nebraska Press.

Eccles, Jacquelynne S., and Bonnie L. Barber. 1999. "Student Council, Volunteering, Basketball, or Marching Band: What Kind of Extracurricular Involvement Matters?" *Journal of Adolescent Research* 14(1):10–43.

Eccles, Jacquelynne S., Carol Freedman-Doan, Pam Frome, Janis Jacobs, and Kwang Suk Yoon. 2000. "Gender-role Socialization in the Family: A Longitudinal Approach." pp. 333–360 in *The Developmental Social Psychology of Gender*, edited by Thomas Eckes and Hannes M. Trautner. Mahwah, NJ: Lawrence Erlbaum.

Eggermant, Steven. 2004. "Television Viewing, Perceived Similarity and Adolescents' Expectations of a Romantic Partner." *Journal of Broadcasting & Electronic Media* 48(2):244–265.

Ekstrom, Mats, and Johan Ostman. 2013. "Family Talk, Peer Talk and Young People's Civic Orientation." *European Journal of Communication* 28(3):294–308.

Ellenwood, Stephan. 2007. "Revisiting Character Education: From McGuffey to Narratives." *Journal of Education* 187(3):21–43.

Elliott, Delbert S., Scott Menard Bruce Rankin, Amanda Elliott, William Julius Wilson, and David Huizinga. 2006. *Good Kids from Bad Neighborhoods: Successful Development in Social Context*. New York: Cambridge University Press.

Elliott, Gregory C., Susan M. Cunningham, Meadow Linder, Melissa Colangelo, and Michelle Gross. 2005. "Child Physical Abuse and Self-perceived Social Isolation among Adolescents." *Journal of Interpersonal Violence* 20(12):1654–1665.

Ellison, Christopher G. 1991. "Identification and Separatism: Religious Involvement and Racial Orientation among Black Americans." *Sociological Quarterly* 22(3):477–494.

Emanuel, A. E. 1990. "Powers in Nonsinusoidal Situations – A Review of Definitions and Physical Meaning." *IEEE Transactions on Power Delivery* 5(3):1377–1389.

Emerson, E., C. Hatton. 2007. "Poverty, Socio-Economic Position, Social Capital and the Health of Children and Adolescents with Intellectual Disabilities in Britain: A Replication." *Journal of Intellectual Disability Research* 51(11):866–874.

Emmanuelle, V. 2009. "Inter-relationships among Attachment to Mother and Father, Self-esteem, and Career Indecision." *Journal of Vocational Behavior* 75(2):91–99.

End, Christian M., Beth Dietz-Uhler, Elizabeth A. Harrick, and Lindy Jacquemotte. 2002. "Identifying with Winners: A Reexamination of Sport Fans' Tendency to BIRG." *Journal of Applied Social Psychology* 32(8):1017–1030.

Engels, Rutger C.M.E., Catrin Finkenauer, Maja Dekovic, and Wim Meeus. 2001. "Parental Attachment and Adolescents' Emotional Adjustment: The Associations with Social Skills and Relevant Competence." *Journal of Counseling Psychology* 48(4):428–439.

Engle, Y., and T. Kasser. 2005. "Why Do Adolescent Girls Idolize Male Celebrities?" *Journal of Adolescent Research* 20(2):263–283.

Englund, Michelle M., Alissa K. Levy, Daniel M. Hyson, and L. Alan Sroufe. 2000. "Adolescent Social Competence: Effectiveness in a Group Setting." *Child Development* 71(4):1049–1060.

Erdley, Cynthia A., and Steven R. Asher. 1996. "Children's Social Goals and Self-efficacy Perceptions as Influences on Their Responses to Ambiguous Provocation." *Child Development* 67:1329–1344.

Erez, Ayelet, Mario Mikulincer, Mrinus H. van Ijzendoon, and Pieter M. Kroonenberg. 2008. "Attachment, Personality and Volunteering: Placing Volunteerism in an Attachment-theoretical Framework." *Personality & Individual Differences* 44:64–74.

Erikson, E. 1950. *Childhood and Society*. New York: Norton.

Erikson, E. H. 1964. "A Memorandum on Identity and Negro Youth." *Journal of Social Issues* 20(4):29–42.

Erikson, E. H. 1968. *Identity: Youth and Crisis*. New York: Norton.

Espelage, Dorothy L., Harold D. Green, Jr., and Stanley Wasserman. 2007. "Statistical Analysis of Friendship Patterns and Bullying Behaviors among Youth." *New Directions for Child & Adolescent Development* 118:61–75.

Eyal, Keren, and René M. Dailey. 2012. "Examining Relational Maintenance in Parasocial Relationships." *Mass Communication & Society* 15(5):758–781.

Eysenck, H. J., and S. B. G. Eysenck. 1975. *Manual of the Eysenck Personality Questionnaire (Junior and Adult)*. Hodder and Stoughton.

Eysenck, S. B., H. J. Eysenck, and P. Barrett. 1985. "A Revised Version of the Psychoticism Scale." *Personality and Individual Differences* 6(1):21–29.

Fahmy, Eldin. 2006. "Social Capital and Civic Action: A Study of Youth in the United Kingdom." *Young* 14(2):101–118.

Fairbrother, Gregory P. 2003. "The Effects of Political Education and Critical Thinking on Hong Kong and Mainland Chinese University Students' National Attitudes." *British Journal of Sociology of Education* 24(5):605–620.

Fairchild, Charles. 2007. "Building the Authentic Celebrity: The Idol Phenomenon in the Attention Economy." *Popular Music & Society* 30(3):355–375.

Faircloth, Beverly S., and Jill V. Hamm. 2005. "Sense of Belonging among High School Students Representing 4 Ethnic Groups." *Journal of Youth & Adolescence* 34(4):293–309.

Falci, Christina, and Clea McNeely. 2009. "Too Many Friends: Social Integration, Network Cohesion and Adolescent Depressive Symptoms." *Social Forces* 87(4):2031–2062.

Farrer, James, and Jeff Gavin. 2009. "Online Dating in Japan: A Test of Social Information Processing Theory." *CyberPsychology & Behavior* 12(4):407–412.

Feeney, J. A., and P. Noller. 1990. "Attachment Style as a Predictor of Adult Romantic Relationships." *Journal of Personality and Social Psychology* 58(2):281.

Feeney, Judith A., Patricia Noller, and Mary Hanrahan. 1994. "Assessing Adult Attachment." pp. 128–152 in *Attachment in Adults: Clinical and Developmental Perspectives*, edited by Michael B. Sperling and William H. Berman. New York: Guilford.

Fein, Melvyn L. 1999. *The Limits of Idealism: When Good Intentions Go Bad*. New York: Kluwer.

Feiring, Candice. 1995. "Concepts of Romance in 15-year-old Adolescents." *Journal of Research on Adolescence* 6(2):181–200.

Feldman, S. Shirley, and Kathryn R. Wentzel. 1995. "Relations of Marital Satisfaction to Peer Outcomes in Adolescent Boys: A Longitudinal Study." *Journal of Early Adolescence* 15(2):226–237.

Feldman, Stanley. 2003. "Enforcing Social Conformity: A Theory of Authoritarianism." *Political Psychology* 24(1):41–74.

Fergusson, D. M., A. L. Beautrais, and L. J. Horwood. 2003. "Vulnerability and Resiliency to Suicidal Behaviors in Young People." *Psychological Medicine* 33:61–73.

Ferris, Kerry O. 2001. "Through a Glass, Darkly: The Dynamics of Fan-celebrity Encounter." *Symbolic Interaction* 24(1):25–47.

Feshbach, S., and B. Weiner. 1986. *Personality*, 2nd ed. Canada: D.C. Health Company.

Fetscherin, Marc, and Santa Barbara. 2014. "What Type of Relationship Do We Have with Loved Brands?" *Journal of Consumer Marketing* 31(6/7):430–440.

Field, T. 1981. "Early Peer Relations." pp. 1–30 in *The utilization of Classroom Peers as Behavior Change Agents*, edited by P. S. Strain. New York: Plenum.

Finkel, Steven E., Howard R. Ernst. 2005. "Civic Education in Post-Apartheid South Africa: Alternative Paths to the Development of Political Knowledge and Democratic Values." *Political Psychology* 26(3):333–364.

Firat, A. Fuat, and Nikhilesch Dholakia. 1998. *Consuming People: From Political Economy to Theaters of Consumption*. London: Routledge.

Flanagan, Constance A., and Bernadette Campbell. 2003. "Social Class and Adolescents' Beliefs about Justice in Different Social Orders." *Journal of Social Issues* 59(4):711–732.

Flannery, Daniel J., Alexander T. Vazsonyi, Julia Torquati, and Angela Fridrich. 1993. "Ethnic and Gender Differences in Risk for Early Adolescent Substance Use." *Journal of Youth & Adolescence* 23(2):195–213.

Fletcher, Annee, Andrea G. Hunter, and Angella Y. Eanes. 2006. "Lines between Social Network Closure and Child Well-being: The Organizing Role of Friendship Context." *Developmental Psychology* 42(6):1057–1068.

Flouri, Eirini, and Ann Buchanan. 2002. "The Protective Role of Parental Involvement in Adolescent Suicide." *Crisis* 23(1):17–22.

Forestier, Katherine, and Michael Crossley. 2015. "International Education Policy Transfer—Borrowing Both Ways: The Hong Kong and England Experience." *Prometheus* 24(4):389–403.

Forman, Tyrone A. 2001. "Social Determinants of White Youths' Racial Attitudes: Evidence from a National Survey." *Sociological Studies of Children and Youth* 8:173–207.

Fortune, Anne E., Alonzo Cavagos, and Mingun Lee. 2005. "Field Education in Social Work Achievement Motivation and Outcome in Social Work Field Education." *Journal of Social Work Education* 41(1):115–129.

Fosco, Gregory M., and Mark E. Feinberg. 2015. "Cascading Effects of Interparental Conflict in Adolescence: Linking Threat Appraisals, Self-Efficacy, and Adjustment." *Development & Psychopathology* 27(1):239–252.

Foster, J. D., M. H. Kernis, and B. M. Goldman. 2007. "Linking Adult Attachment to Self-esteem Stability." *Self and Identity* 6(1):64–73.

Franco, Zeno E., Kathy Blau, and Philip G. Zimbardo. 2011. "Heroism: A conceptual analysis and differentiation between heroic action and altruism." *Review of General Psychology* 15(2):99–113.

Franklin, Maureen. 1995. "The Effects of Differential College Environments on Academic Learning and Student Perceptions of Cognitive Development." *Research in Higher Education* 36(2):127–153.

Fraser, Benson P., and William J. Brown. 2002. "Media, Celebrities, and Social Influence: Identification with Elvis Presley." *Mass Communication & Society* 5(2):183–206.

Fredricks, Jennifer A., and Jacquelynne S. Eccles. 2005. "Developmental Benefits of Extracurricular Involvement: Do Peer Characteristics Mediate the Link between Activities and Youth Outcomes?" *Journal of Youth & Adolescence* 34(6):507–520.

Freeman, Harry, and B. Bradford Brown. 2001. "Primary Attachment to Parents and Peers during Adolescence: Differences by Attachment Style." *Journal of Youth & Adolescence* 30(6):653–674.

Freud, S. 1925. "Negation." *The International Journal of Psycho-Analysis* 6:367.

Freud, S. 1951. *Group Psychology and the Analysis of the Ego*, edited and translated by J. Strachey. New York: Liveright (original work published 1922).

Frith, Simon. 1983. *Sound Effects: Youth, Leisure, and the Politics of Rock*. London: Constable, 202–234.

Froiland, John Mark, Paivi Mayor, and Marjaana Herlevi. 2015. "Motives Emanating from Personality Associated with Achievement in a Finnish Senior High School: Physical Activity, Curiosity, and Family Motives." *School Psychology International* 36(2):207–221.

Fromm, E. (1967). *On Being Human*. London: A&C Black.

Furman, Wyndol, and Jessica K. Winkles. 2010. "Predicting Romantic Involvement, Relationship Cognitions, and Relationship Qualities from Physical Appearance,

Perceived Norms, and Relational Styles Regarding Friends and Parents." *Journal of Adolescence* 33:827–836.

Furnham, Adrian. 1990. *The Protestant Work Ethic: The Psychology of Work-Related Beliefs and Behaviors.* London: Routledge.

Furnham-Diggory, Syliva. 1992. *Cognitive Process in Education.* New York: HarperCollins.

Galambos, Nancy L., Sheria A. Berenbaum, and Susan M. McHale. 2009. "Gender Development in Adolescence." pp. 305–357 in *Handbook of Adolescent Psychology*, 3rd ed., Vol. 1, edited by Richard M. Lerner and Laurence Steinberg. Hoboken, NJ: Wiley.

Gamble, Andrew. 2010. "Ethics and Politics." pp. 73–89 in *Ethics and World Politics*, edited by Duncan Bell. Oxford, UK: Oxford University Press.

Gambrill, Eileen. 2005. *Critical Thinking in Clinical Practice: Improving the Quality of Judgments and Decisions.* Hoboken, NJ: Wiley.

Gangestad, Steven W., Martie G. Haselton, and David M. Buss. 2006. "Evolutionary Foundations of Cultural Variation: Evoked Culture and Mate Preferences." *Psychological Inquiry* 17(2):75–95.

Garcia, Jeanette M., John R. Sirard, Nancy L. Deutsch, and Arthur Weltman. 2016. "The Influence of Friends and Psychosocial Factors on Physical Activity and Screen Time Behavior in Adolescents: A Mixed-Methods Analysis." *Journal of Behavioral Medicine* 39(4):610–623.

Garratt, Sheryl. [1984] 1990. "Teenage Dreams." pp. 399–409 in *On Record: Rock, Pop, and the Written Word*, edited by Simon Frith and Andrew Goodwin. London: Routledge.

Gash, H., M. Morgan, and C. Sugrue. 1993. "Modifying Gender Stereotypes in Primary School." *The Irish Journal of Education/Iris Eireannach an Oideachais* 27(1/2):60–70.

Gash, Hugh, and Paul Conway. 1997. "Images of Heroes and Heroines: How Stable?" *Journal of Applied Developmental Psychology* 18:349–372.

Georgas, Tames, Sophia Christakopoalou, Ype H. Poortinga, Alois Ahgleitner, Robin Goodwin, and Neophytos Charalambous. 1997. "The Relationship of Family Bonds to Family Structure and Function across Cultures." *Journal of Cross-Cultural Psychology* 28(3):303–320.

Gershuny, Jonathan. 2000. *Changing Times: Work and Leisure in Postindustrial Society.* Oxford, UK: Oxford University Press.

Giancarlo, Carol Ann, and Peter A. Facione. 2001. "A Look across Four Years at the Disposition toward Critical Thinking among Undergraduate Students." *Journal of General Education* 50(1):29–55.

Gibbs, John C., Karen S. Basinger, Rebecca L. Grime, and John R. Snarey. 2007. "Moral Judgment Development across Cultures: Revisiting Kohlberg's Universality Claims." *Developmental Review* 27(4):443–500.

Gibson, Diane. 2001. "Food Stamp Program Participation and Health: Estimates for the NLSY97." pp. 258–295 in *Social Awakening: Adolescent Behavior as Adulthood Approaches*, edited by Robert T. Michael. New York: Russell Sage.

Giles, D. C., and J. Maltby. 2004. "The Role of Media Figures in Adolescent Development: Relations between Autonomy, Attachment, and Interest in Celebrities." *Personality and Individual Differences* 36(4):813–822.

Giles, David. 2000. *Illusions of Immortality: A Psychology of Fame and Celebrity.* Houndmills, UK: Macmillan.

Gillath, Omri, Phillip R. Shaver, Mario Mikulineer, Rachel E. Nitzberg, Ayelet Erez, and Marinus H. van Izendoorr. 2005. "Attachment, Caregiving, and Volunteering: Placing Volunteerism in an Attachment-Theoretical Framework." *Personal Relationships* 12:425–466.

Giordano, Peggy C., Monica A. Longore, and Wendy D. Manning. 2001. "On the Nature and Developmental Significance of Adolescent Romantic Relationships." *Sociological Studies of Children and Youth* 8:111–139.

Giordano, Peggy C., Monica A. Longmore, Ryan D. Schroeder, and Patrick M. Seffrin. 2008. "A Life-course Perspective on Spirituality and Desistance from Crime." *Criminology* 46(1):99–132.

Girsh, Yaron. 2014. "Between My Mother and the Big Brother: Israeli Adolescents' Views of Heroes and Celebrities." *Journal of Youth Studies* 17(7):916–929.

Glanville, Jennifer L., David Sikkink, and Edwin I. Harnandez. 2008. "Religious Involvement and Educational Outcomes: The Role of Social Capital and Extracurricular Participation." *Sociological Quarterly* 49:105–137.

Glatz, Terese, and Viktor Dahl. 2014. "The Role of Family Experiences for Adolescents' Readiness to Use and Participate in Illegal Political Activity." *International Journal of Behavioral Development* 40(1):11–20.

Gleason, Tracy R., Sally A. Theran, and Emily M. Newberg. 2017. "Parasocial Interactions and Relationships in Early Adolescence." *Frontiers in Psychology* 8:255.

Glennie, Paul. 1998. "Consumption, Consumerism, and Urban Form: Historical Perspectives." *Urban Studies* 35(5/6):927–951.

Goethals, George R., and Scott T. Allison. 2012. "Making Heroes: The Construction of Courage, Competence, and Virtue." *Advances in Experimental Social Psychology* 46:183–235.

Goldberg, L. R., and T. K. Rosolack. 1994. "The Big Five Factor Structure as an Integrative Framework: An Empirical Comparison with Eysenck's PEN Model." *The Developing Structure of Temperament and Personality from Infancy to Adulthood*: 7–35.

Gomez, R., and S. McLaren. 2007. The Inter-relations of Mother and Father Attachment, Self-esteem and Aggression during Late Adolescence." *Aggressive Behavior* 33(2):160–169.

Gonzalez, Oscar I., Raymond W. Novaco, Mark A. Reger, and Gregory A. Gahm. 2016. "Anger Intensification with Combat-Related PTSD and Depression Comorbidity." *Psychological Trauma: Theory, Research, Practice, & Policy* 8(1):9–16.

Gore, Susan, and Robert H. Aseltine, Jr. 1995. "Protective Processes in Adolescence: Matching Stressors with Social Resources." *American Journal of Community Psychology* 23(3):301–327.

Gormley, William T., Jr., Ted Gayer, Deborah Phillips, and Brittany Dawson. 2005. "The Effects of Universal Pre-K on Cognitive Development." *Developmental Psychology* 41(6):872–884.

Goss, David. 2005. "Entrepreneurship and the Social: Towards a Deference-emotion Theory." *Human Relations* 58(5):617–636.

Gottfried, Michael A. 2013. "The Spillover Effects of Grade-Retained Classmates: Evidence from Urban Elementary Schools." *American Journal of Education* 119(3):405–444.

Gountas, John, Sandra Gountas, Robert A. Reeves, and Lucy Moran. 2012. "Desire for Fame: Scale Development and Association with Personal Goals and Aspirations." *Psychology & Marketing* 29(9):680–689.

Graham, Christine A., and M. Ann Easterbrooks. 2000. "School-aged Children, Vulnerability to Depressive Symptomatology: The Role of Attachment Security, Maternal Depressive Symptomatology, and Economic Risk." *Development & Psychopathology* 12:201–213.

Granqvist, P. 1998. "Religiousness and Perceived Childhood Attachment: On the Question of Compensation or Correspondence." *Journal for the Scientific Study of Religion* 37(2):350–367.

Granqvist, Pehr, and Jane R. Dickie. 2005. "Attachment and Spiritual Development in Childhood and Adolescence." pp. 197–210 in *The Handbook of Spiritual Development in Childhood and Adolescence*, edited by Eugene C. Roehlkepartain, Pamela Ebstyne King, Linda Wagener, and Peter L. Benson. Thousand Oaks, CA: Sage.

Grasmick, Harold G., John Hagan, Brenda Sims Blackwell, and Bruce J. Arneklev. 1996. "Risk Preferences and Patriarchy: Extending Power-control Theory." *Social Forces* 75(1):177–199.

Greenberg, Jeff, Spee Kosloff, Sheldon Solomon, Florette Cohen, and Mark Landau. 2010. "Toward Understanding the Fame Game: The Effect of Mortality Salience on the Appeal of Fame." *Self & Identity* 9(1):1–18.

Greene, A. L., and Carolyn Adams-Price. 1990. "Adolescents' Secondary Attachments to Celebrity Figures." *Sex Roles* 23:335–347.

Greenwood, Dara N. 2007. "Are Female Action Heroes Risky Role Models? Character Identification, Idealization, and Viewer Aggression." *Sex Roles* 57(9–10):725–732.

Greenwood, Dara N., and Christopher R. Long. 2011. "Attachment, Belongingness Needs, and Relationship." *Communication Research* 38(2):278–297.

Greeson, L. E., and R. A. Williams. 1986. "Social Implications of Music Videos for Youth: An Analysis of the Content and Effects of MTV." *Youth & Society* 18:177–189.

Griffin, Kenneth W., Gilbert J. Botvin, Lawrence M. Scheier, Tracy Diaz, and Nicole L. Miller. 2000. "Parenting Practices as Predictors of Substance Use, Delinquency, and Aggression among Urban Minority Youth: Moderating Effects of Family Structure and Gender." *Psychology of Addictive Behaviors* 14(2):174–184.

Grunebaum, James O. 2003. *Friendship: Liberty, Equality, and Utility.* Albany, NY: State University of New York Press.

Grych, John H., and Kristen M. Kinsfogel. 2010. "Exploring the Role of Attachment Style in the Relation between Family Aggression and Abuse in Adolescent Dating Relationships." *Journal of Aggression, Maltreatment & Trauma* 19(6):624–640.

Guay, Frederic, Catherine F. Ratelle, Caroline Senecal, Simon Larose, and Andree Deschenes. 2006. "Distinguishing Developmental from Chronic Career Indecision: Self-efficacy, Autonomy, and Social Support." *Journal of Career Assessment* 14(2):235–251.

Gullone, Elenoru, Thomas H. Ollendick, and Neville J. King. 2006. "The Role of Attachment Representation in the Relationship between Symptomatology and School Withdrawal in Middle Childhood." *Journal of Child & Family Studies* 15(3):271–285.

Gummerum, Michaela, and Monika Keller. 2008. "Affection, Virtue, Pleasure, and profit: Developing an Understanding of Friendship Closeness and Intimacy in Western and Asian Societies." *International Journal of Behavioral Development* 32(3):218–231.

Haas, Anne, and Stanford W. Gregory, Jr. 2005. "The Impact of Physical Attractiveness on Women's Social Status and Interactional Power." *Sociological Forum* 20(3):449–469.

Hafner, Michael. 2009. "Knowing You, Knowing Me: Familiarity Moderates Comparison Outcomes to Idealized Media Images." *Social Cognition* 27(4):496–508.

Hagan, John, and Holly Foster. 2001. "Youth Violence and the End of Adolescence." *American Sociological Review* 66:874–899.

Hakim, Catherine. 2010. "Erotic Capital." *European Sociological Review* 26(5):499–518.

Hallett, Tim. 2007. "Between Defence and Distinction: Interaction Ritual through Symbolic Power in an Educational Institution." *Social Psychology Quarterly* 70(2):148–171.

Halpern, Carslyn Tucker, Rosalind Berkowitz King, Selene G. Osak, and J. Richard Udry. 2005. "Body Mass Index, Dieting, Romance, and Sexual Activity in Adolescent Girls: Relationships over Time." *Journal of Research on Adolescence* 15(4):535–559.

Halpern, D. F. 1998. "Teaching Critical Thinking for Transfer across Domains: Disposition, Skills, Structure Training, and Metacognitive Monitoring." *American Psychologist* 53(4):449.

Hamilton, S. F., and N. Darling. 1996. "Mentors in Adolescents' Lives." *Social Problems and Social Context in Adolescence: Perspectives across Boundaries,* edited by Klaus Hurrelmann and Stephen F. Hamlton. New York: Aldine de Gruyer.

Hamilton, Vivian E. 2010. "Immature Citizens and the State." *Brigham Young University Law Review* 2010(4):1055–1147.

Hand, Matthew M., Donna Thomas, Walter C. Buboltz, Eric D. Deemer, and Munkhsanaa Buyanjargal. 2013. "Facebook and Romantic Relationships: Intimacy and Couple Satisfaction Associated with Online Social Network Use." *Cyberpsychology, Behavior & Social Networking* 16(1):8–13.

Hansell, Stephen, and Helene Raskin White. 1991. "Adolescent Drug Use, Psychological Distress, and Physical Symptoms." *Journal of Health and Social Behavior* 32:288–301.

Hao, Lingxin, and Melissa Bonstead-Bruns. 1998. "Parent-child Differences in Educational Expectations and the Academic Achievement of Immigrant and Native Students." *Sociology of Education* 71:175–198.

Harter, Susan. 2012. *The Construction of the Self: Developmental and Sociocultural Foundations.* New York: Guilford.

Hartup, William W. 1996. "The Company They Keep: Friendships and Their Developmental Significance." *Child Development* 67:1–13.

Hay, Carter. 2001. "An Exploratory Test of Braithwaite's Reintegrative Shaming Theory." *Journal of Research in Crime and Delinquency* 38(2):132–153.

Hay, Carter. 2003. "Family Strain, Gender, and Delinquency." *Sociological Perspectives* 46(1):107–130.

Haynie, Dana L. 2001. "Delinquent Peers Revisited: Does Network Structure Matter?" *American Journal of Sociology* 106(4):1013–1057.

He, Xiaozhong. 2006. "Survey Report on Idol Worship among Children and Young People." *Chinese Education & Society* 39(1):84–103.

He, Yuzhang, and Xiaotian Feng. 2002. "Idol Worship amongst the Youth: A Sociological Analysis of 207 Letters from Zhao Wei Fans." *Chinese Education & Society* 35(6):81–94.

Heffernan, Troy, Mark Morrison, Parikshit Basu, and Arthur Sweeney. 2010. "Cultural Differences, Learning Styles and Transnational Education." *Journal of Higher Education Policy & Management* 32(1):27–39.

Hellevik, Tale, and Richard A. Settersten, Jr. 2013. "Life Planning among Young Adults in 23 European Countries: The Effects of Individual and Country Security." *European Sociological Review* 29(5):923–938.

Helwig, Andrew A. 2004. "A Ten-year Longitudinal Study of the Career Development of Students: Summary Findings." *Journal of Counseling & Development* 82:49–57.

Henderson, Craig E., Bert Hayslip, Jr., Leah M. Sanders, and Linda Louden. 2009. "Grandmother-grandchild Relationship Quality Predicts Psychological Adjustment among Youth from Divorced Families." *Journal of Family Issues* 30(9):1245–1264.

Hendry, Leo B., Janet Shucksmith, John G. Love, and Anthony Glendinning. 1993. *Young People's Leisure and Lifestyles.* London: Routledge.

Henry, Rachael M. 1983. *The Psychodynamic Foundations of Morality.* Basel, Switzerland: Karger.

Hickman, Gregory P., Suanne Bartholomae, and Patrick C. McKenry. 2000. "Influence of Parenting Styles on the Adjustment and Academic Achievement of Traditional College Freshmen." *Journal of College Student Development* 41(1):41–54.

Hill, Roger B., and Jay W. Rojewski. 1999. "Double Jeopardy: Work Ethic Differences in Youth at Risk of School Failure." *Career Development Quarterly* 47:267–280.

Hirschi, Andreas. 2009. "Career Adaptability Development in Adolescence: Multiple Predictors and Effects on Sense of Power and Life Satisfaction." *Journal of Vocational Behavior* 74:145–155.

Ho, K. L. 2008. *Parental Styles, Idol Worship and Self Efficacy: A Study among 205 Hong Kong Secondary School and University Students.* Undergraduate Thesis, City University of Hong Kong.

Hocking, Elise C., Raluca M. Simons, and Renata J. Surette. 2016. "Attachment Style as a Mediator between Childhood Maltreatment and the Experience of Betrayal Trauma as an Adult." *Child Abuse & Neglect* 52:94–101.

Hoegele, Daniel, Sascha L. Schmidt, and Benno Torgler. 2014. "Superstars as Drivers of Organizational Identification: Empirical Findings from Professional Soccer." *Psychology & Marketing* 31(9):736–757.

Hoegh, Dana G., and Martin Bourgeois. 2002. "Prelude and Postlude to the Self: Correlates of Achieved Identity." *Youth & Society* 33(4):573–594.

Hoffman, Dylan. 2014. "Becoming Beautiful: The Aesthetics of Individuation." *Psychological Perspectives* 57(1):50–64.

Hoffman, Martin L. 2000. *Empathy and Moral Development: Implications for Caring and Justice.* Cambridge, UK: Cambridge University Press.

Holland, Alyce, and Thomas Andre. 1987. "Participation in Extracurricular Activities in Secondary School: What Is Known, What Needs to Be Known?" *Review of Educational Research* 57(4, Winter):437–466.

Holt, Douglas B. 1997. "Poststructuralist Lifestyle Analysis: Conceptualizing the Social Patterning of Consumption in Postmodernity." *Journal of Consumer Research* 23:326–350.

Holub, Shayla C., Marie S. Tisak, and David Mullins. 2008. "Gender Differences in Children's Hero Attributions: Personal Hero Choices and Evaluations of Typical Male and Female Heroes." *Sex Roles* 58(7–8):567–578.

Hooghe, Marc, Ruth Dassonneville, and Sofie Marien. 2015. "The Impact of Education on the Development of Political Trust: Results from a Five-Year Panel Study among Late Adolescents and Young Adults in Belgium." *Political Studies* 63(1):123–141.

Hoover, M., and L. O. Stokes. 2003. "Hong Kong in New York: Global Connections, National Identity, and Film Representations." *New Political Science* 25:509–532.

Hou, W., Y. Zhang, and M. Huang. 2003. *Conflict and Integration.* Beijing, China: Chinese People University Press.

Houran, James, Samir Navik, and Keeli Zerrusen. 2005. "Boundary Functioning in Celebrity Worshippers." *Personality & Individual Differences* 38:237–248.

Hsiao, Yangji. 2004. Shaping Modern Citizens: Study of the Development and Cultivation of Senior Secondary Student Citizenship. Taipei, Taiwan: Weber Culture.

Huang, Hazel H., and Vincent-Wayne Mitchell. 2014. "The Role of Imagination and Brand Personification in Brand Relationships." *Psychology & Marketing* 31(1):38–47.

Huang, Ji. 1998. *General Theory of Educational Philosophy.* Taiyuan, China: Shanxi Educational.

Huang, Ya-Rong. 2006. "Identity and Intimacy Crises and Their Relationship to Internet Dependence among College Students." *Cyber Psychology & Behavior* 9(5):571–576.

Hudders, Liselot, and Mario Pandelaere. 2012. "The Silver Lining of Materialism: The Impact of Luxury Consumption on Substance Well-being." *Journal of Happiness Studies* 13:411–437.

Huebner, Angela J., and Sherry C. Betts. 2002. "Exploring the Utility of Social Control Theory for Youth Development: Issues of Attachment, Involvement, and Gender." *Youth & Society* 34(2):123–145.

Hurd, Noelle M., Marc A. Zimmerman, and Thomas M. Reischl. 2011. "Role Model Behavior and Youth Violence: A Study of Positive and Negative Effects." *Journal of Early Adolescence* 31(2):323–354.

Hwang, Keumjoong. 2013. "Educational Modes of Thinking in Neo-Confucianism: A Traditional Lens for Rethinking Modern Education." *Asia Pacific Education Review* 14(2):243–253.

Ibarra, Peter R., and John I. Kitsuse. 2003. "Claims-making Discourse and Vernacular Resources." pp. 17–50 in *Challenges and Choices: Constructionist Perspectives on*

Social Problems, edited by James A. Holstein and Gale Miller. New York: Aldine de Gruyter.

Ickes, William, Anna Park, and Amanda Johnson. 2012. "Linking Identity Status to Strength of Sense of Self: Theory and Validation." *Self & Identity* 11(4):531–544.

Ikels, Charlotte. 1989. "Becoming a Human Being in Theory and Practice: Chinese Views of Human Development." pp. 109–134 in *Age Structuring in Comparative Perspective*, edited by David I. Kertzer and K. Warner Schaie. Hillsdale, NJ: Lawrence Erlbaum Associates.

Irazabal, Clara, and Surajit Chakravarty. 2007. "Entertainment-retail Centres in Hong Kong and Los Angeles: Trends and Lessons." *International Planning Studies* 12(3):241–271.

Ivaldi, Antonia, and Susan A. O'Neill. 2008. "Adolescents' Musical Role Models: Whom Do They Admire and Why?" *Psychology of Music* 36(4):395–415.

Jackson, Linda A., Alexander von Eye, Frank A. Brocca, Gretchen Babatsis, and Yong Zhao. 2006. "Does Home Internet Use Influence the Academic Performance of Low-income Children?" *Developmental Psychology* 42(3):429–435.

Jakoubek, Jane, and Robyn R. Swenson. 1993. "Differences in Use of Learning Strategies and Relation to Grades among Undergraduate Students." *Psychological Report* 73:787–793.

Jang, Sung Joon. 1999. "Age-varying Effects of Family, School and Peers on Delinquency: A Multilevel Modeling Test of Interactional Theory." *Criminology* 37(3):643–685.

Jang, Sung Joon, and Aaron B. Franzen. 2013. "Is Being Spiritual Enough without Being Religious? A Study of Violent and Property Crimes among Emerging Adults." *Criminology* 51(3):595–627.

Janssens, Jan M. A. M., and Maja Dekovic. 1997. "Child Rearing, Prosocial Moral Reasoning and Prosocial Behavior." *International Journal of Behavioral Development* 20(3):509–527.

Jeffrey, A. 1991. "Adolescents and Heavy Metal Music." *Journal of Youth and Society* 23:76–98.

Jenson, Joli. 1992. "Fandom as Pathology: The Consequences of Characterization." pp. 9–29 in *The Adoring Audience: Fan Culture and Popular Media*, edited by Lisa A. Lewis. London: Routledge.

Jessor, Richard, Marks Turbin, Frances M. Costa, Qi Dong, Hong Chuan Zhang, and Changhai Wang. 2003. "Adolescent Problem Behavior in China and the United States: A Cross-national Study of Psychosocial Protection Factors." *Journal of Research in Adolescence* 13(3):329–360.

Jiang, Binghai, Keqian Wang, Huajin Zhang, Zhaoyi Jiang, and Kun Xu. 1993. *Introduction to Spiritual Civilization*. Shanghai, China: Shanghai People's.

Jiang, Xu, E. Scott Huebner, and Kimberly J. Hills. 2013. "Parent Attachment and Early Adolescents' Life Satisfaction: The Mediating Effect of Hope." *Psychology in the Schools* 50(4):340–352.

Jiang, Yi, Mimi Bong, and Sung-il Kim. 2015. "Conformity of Korean Adolescents in Their Perceptions of Social Relationships and Academic Motivation." *Learning & Individual Differences* 40:41–54.

Jin, Yuchang, Cuicui Sun, Junxiu An, and Junyi Li. 2017. "Attachment Styles and Smartphone Addiction in Chinese College Students: The Mediating Roles of Dysfunctional Attitudes and Self-Esteem." *International Journal of Mental Health & Addiction* 15(5):1122–1134.

Jing, Huaibin, Chen Zheng, and Haipeng Xiao. 1995. "People's Cultural Momentum and Modernization: Report of the Study of the Cultural Momentum of Urban Residents in China." Beijing, China: People's.

Job, J. G. 2002. "Young Love." *Parents* 77(2):145–146.

Johnson, David W., and Roger T. Johnson. 1993. "Creative and Critical Thinking through Academic Controversy." *American Behavioral Scientist* 37(1):40–53.

Johnson, Laura R., Julie S. Johnson-Pynn, Thomas M. Pynn. 2007. "Youth Civic Engagement in China's Results from a Program Promoting Environmental Activism." *Journal of Adolescent Research* 22(4):355–386.

Johnson, Sara K., Mary H. Buckingham, Stacy L. Morris, Sara Suzuki, Michelle B. Weiner, Rachel M. Hershberg, Ettya R. Fremont, Milena Batanova, Caitlin C. Aymong, Cristina J. Hunter, Edmond P. Bowers, Jacqueline V. Lerner, and Richard M. Lerner. 2016. "Adolescents' Character Role Models: Exploring Who Young People Look Up to as Examples of How to Be a Good Person." *Research in Human Development* 13(2):126–141.

Johnston, Kim L., and Katherine M. White, 2003. "Binge-Drinking: A Test of the Role of Group Norms in the Theory of Planned Behaviour." *Psychology & Health* 18(1):63–77.

Jones, Caria E., and John D. Watt. 1999. "Psychosocial Development and Moral Orientation among Traditional-aged College Students." *Journal of College Student Development* 40(2):125–131.

Jones, David W. 2016. *Disordered Personalities and Crime: An Analysis of the History of Moral Insanity.* Abingdon, UK: Routledge.

Joseph, Pamela Bolotin, and Sara Efron. 2005. "Seven Worlds of Moral Education." *Phi Delta Kappan* 86(7):525–533.

Josselson, R. 1991. *Finding Herself: Pathways to Identity Development in Women.* San Francisco, CA: Jossey-Bass.

Julal, F. S., K. B. Carnelley, and A. Rowe. 2017. "The Relationship between Attachment Style and Placement of Parents in Adults' Attachment Networks over Time." *Attachment & Human Development* 19(4):382–406.

Kahne, Joseph, and Ellen Middaugh. 2009. "Democracy for Some: The Civic Opportunity Gap in High School." pp. 29–58 in *Engaging Young People in Civic Life*, edited by James Youniss and Peter Levine. Nashville, TN: Vanderbilt University Press.

Kahne, Joseph, Bernadette Chi, and Ellen Middaugh. 2006. "Building Social Capital for Civic and Political Engagement: The Potential of High-school Civics Courses." *Canadian Journal of Education* 29(2):387–409.

Kahne, Joseph, Nam-Jin Lee, and Jessica T. Feezell. 2013a. "The Civic and Political Significance of Online Participatory Cultures among Youth Transitioning to Adulthood." *Journal of Information Technology & Politics* 10(1):1–20.

Kalczynski, Paul A., James M. Fauth, and Amy Swanger. 1998. "Adolescent Identity: Rational vs. Experiential Processing, Formal Operations, and Critical Thinking Beliefs." *Journal of Youth & Adolescence* 27(2):185–207.

Kam, Chui Ping Iris. 2012. "Personal Identity versus National Identity among Hong Kong Youths: Personal and Social Education Reform after Reunification." *Social Identities* 18(6):649–661.

Kam, W. K. 2013. *Idol Worship, Personality and Self-Esteem.* Undergraduate Thesis, City University of Hong Kong.

Kamptner, N. L. 1988. "Identity Development in Late Adolescence: Causal Modeling of Social and Familial Influence." *Journal of Youth & Adolescence* 17:493–514.

Kaplan E. Joseph, and Daniel A. Kies. 1994. "Strategies to Increase Critical Thinking in the Undergraduate College Classroom." *College Student Journal* 28(1):24–31.

Kappes, Heather Barry, Bettina Schwörer, and Gabriele Oettingen. 2012. "Needs Instigate Positive Fantasies of Idealized Futures." *European Journal of Social Psychology* 42(3):299–307.

Karniol, Rachel. 2001. "Adolescent Females' Idolization of Male Media Stars as a Transition into Sexuality." *Sex Roles* 44(1/2):61–77.

Kasen, Stephanie, Kathy Berenson, Patricia Cohen, and Jeffrey G. Johnson. 2004. "The Effects of School Climate on Changes in Aggressive and Other Behaviors Related to Bullying." pp. 189–210 in *Bullying in American Schools: A Social-ecological Perspective on Prevention and Intervention*, edited by Dorothy L. Espelage and Susan M. Swearer. Mahwah, NJ: Lawrence Erlbaum.

Katz-Wise, Sabra L., Stephanie L. Budge, Sara M. Lindberg, and Janet S. Hyde. 2013. "Individuation or Identification? Self-Objectification and the Mother-Adolescent Relationship." *Psychology of Women Quarterly* 37(3):366–380.

Kawamura, Yuniya. 2006. "Japanese Teens as Producers of Street Fashion." *Current Sociology* 54(5):784–801.

Kegler, Michelle Crozier, Roy F. Oman, Sara K. Veskly, Kenneth R. McLeroy, Cheryl B. Aspy, Sharon Rodine, and La Donna Marshall. 2005. "Relationships among Youth Assets and Neighborhood and Community Resources." *Health Education & Behavior* 32(3):380–397.

Keller, Joshua, and Jeffrey Loewenstein. 2011. "The Cultural Category of Cooperation: A Cultural Consensus Model Analysis for China and the United States." *Organization Science* 22(2):299–319.

Kelly, Erin L., Phyllis Moen, and Eric Tranby. 2011. "Changing Workplaces to Reduce Work-family Conflict, Schedule Central in a White-collar Organization." *American Sociological Review* 76(2):265–290.

Kennedy, Janice H. 1999. "Romantic Attachment Style and Ego Identity, Attributional Style, and Family of Origin in First-year College Students." *College Student Journal* 33(2):171–180.

Kezar, Adrianna, and Deb Moriarty. 2000. "Expanding Our Understanding of Student Leadership Development: A Study Exploring Gender and Ethnic Identity." *Journal of College Student Development* 41(1):55–69.

Kim, Young-Il, and W. Bradford Wilcox. 2013. "Bonding Alone: Familism, Religion, and Secular Civic Participation." *Social Science Research* 42(1):31–45.

King, Pamela Ebstyne. 2007. "Adolescent Spirituality and Positive Youth Development: A Look at Religion, Social Capital and Moral Functioning." pp. 227–242 in *Approaches to Positive Youth Development*, edited by Rainer K. Silbereisen and Richard M. Lerner. Thousand Oaks, CA: Sage.

King, Pamela Ebstyne, and James L. Furrow. 2004. "Religion as a Resource for Positive Youth Development: Religion, Social Capital, and Moral Outcomes." *Developmental Psychology* 40(5):703–713.

King, Pamela Ebstyne, and Peter L. Benson. 2005. "Spiritual Developmental and Adolescent Well-being and Thriving." pp. 384–398 in *The Handbook of Spiritual Development in Childhood and Adolescence*, edited by Eugene C. Roehlkepartain, Pamela Ebstyne King, Linda Wagener, and Peter L. Benson. Thousand Oaks, CA: Sage.

King, Pamela Ebstyne, and Robert W. Roeser. 2009. "Religion and Spirituality in Adolescent Development." pp. 435–478 in *Handbook of Adolescent Psychology*, 3rd ed. Vol. 1, edited by Richard M. Lerner and Laurence Steinberg. Hoboken, NJ: Wiley.

Kinsella, Elaine L., Timothy D. Ritchie, and Eric R. Igou. 2015a. "Lay Perspectives on the Social and Psychological Functions of Heroes." *Frontiers in Psychology* 6:130.

Kinsella, Elaine L., Timothy D. Ritchie, and Eric R. Igou. 2015b. "Zeroing in on Heroes: A Prototype Analysis of Hero Features." *Journal of Personality and Social Psychology: Personality Processes and Individual Differences* 108(1):114–127.

Kirk, David S. 2009. "Unraveling the Contextual Effects on Student Suspension and Juvenile Arrest: The Independent and Interdependent Influences of School, Neighborhood, and Family Social Controls." *Criminology* 47(2):479–520.

Kirkpatrick, L. A. 1997. "A Longitudinal Study of Changes in Religious Belief and Behavior as a Function of Individual Differences in Adult Attachment Style." *Journal for the Scientific Study of Religion* 36(2):207–217.

Kirkpatrick, L. A. 1999. "Attachment and Religious Representations and Behavior." pp. 803–822 in *Handbook of Attachment: Theory, Research, and Clinical Applications*. New York: Guilford Press.

Kirkpatrick, L. A., and P. R. Shaver. 1990. "Attachment Theory and Religion: Childhood Attachments, Religious Beliefs, and Conversion." *Journal for the Scientific Study of Religion* 29(3): 315–334.

Kirkpatrick, L. A., and P. R. Shaver. 1992. "An Attachment—Theoretical Approach to Romantic Love and Religious Belief." *Personality and Social Psychology Bulletin* 18(3):266–275.

Kirsh, Steven J. 2010. *Media and Youth: A Developmental Perspective.* Chichester, UK: Wiley.

Koh, Caroline, Woon Chia Liu, Stefanie Chye, and Shanti Divaharan. 2013. "Student Teachers' Views on National Education: The Need for Greater Alignment between Policy and Praxis." *Asia Pacific Journal of Education* 33(4):424–443.

Konijn, Elly A., Marjie Nije Bijvank, and Brad J. Bushman. 2007. "I Wish I Were a Warrior: The Role of Wishful Identification and Effects of Violent Video Games on Aggression in Adolescent Boys." *Developmental Psychology* 43(4):1038–1044.

Korobov, Neill. 2004. "Inoculating against Prejudice: A Discursive Approach to Homophobia and Sexism in Adolescent Male Talk." *Psychological of Men & Masculinity* 5(2):178–189.

Kramer, Deiradre A., and Jacqueline Melchoir. 1990. "Gender, Role Conflict, and the Development of Relativistic and Dialectical Thinking." *Sex Roles* 23(9/10):553–575.

Krauss, Steven Eric, Jessica Collura, Shepherd Zeldin, Adriana Ortega, Haslinda Abdullah, and Abdul Hadi Sulaiman. 2014. "Youth-adult Partnership: Exploring Contribution to Empowerment, Agency and Community Connections in Malaysia Youth Programs." *Journal of Youth & Adolescence* 43:1550–1562.

Kristjansson, Kristjan. 2006. "Emulation and the Use of Role Models in Moral Education." *Journal of Moral Education* 35(1):37–49.

Kroger, J. 1996. *Identity in Adolescence: The Balance between Self and Other*, 2nd ed. London: Routledge.

Kruse, Joachim, and Sabine Walper. 2008. "Types of Individuation in Relation to Parents: Predictors and Outcomes." *International Journal of Behavioral Development* 32(5):390–400.

Kuah-Pearce, Kuhn Eng, and Yiu Chak Fong. 2010. "Identity and Sense of Belonging in Post-Colonial Education in Hong Kong." *Asia Pacific Journal of Education* 30(4):433–448.

La Guardia, Jennifer G., Richard M. Ryan, Charles E. Couchman, and Edward L. Deci. 2000. "Within-person Variation in Security of Attachment: A Within-person Variation in Security of Attachment: A Self-determination Theory Perspective on Attachment, Need, Fulfillment, and Well-being." *Journal of Personality & Social Psychology* 79(3):367–384.

Lai, Pak-Sang, and Michael Begram. 2003. "The Politics of Bilingualism: A Reproduction Analysis of the Policy of Mother Tongue Education in Hong Kong after 1997." *Compare* 33(3):315–334.

Laible, D. J., G. Carlo, and S. C. Roesch. 2004. "Pathways to Self-esteem in Late Adolescence: The Role of Parent and Peer Attachment, Empathy, and Social Behaviours." *Journal of Adolescence* 27(6):703–716.

Lam, T. H., S. M. Stewart, and L. M. Ho. 2001. "Smoking and High-risk Sexual Behavior among Young Adults in Hong Kong." *Journal of Behavioral Medicine* 24(5):503–518.

Lapsley, D. K., K. G. Rice, and D. P. FitzGerald. 1990. "Adolescent Attachment, Identity, and Adjustment to College: Implications for the Continuity of Adaptation Hypothesis." *Journal of Counseling & Development* 68(5):561–565.

Lapsley, Daniel K. 1996. "Moral Psychology." Boulder, CO: Westview.

Lapsley, Daniel K., and Jason Edgerton. 2002. "Separation-individuation, Adult Attachment Style, and College Adjustment." *Journal of Counseling & Development* 80(4):484–492.

Larose, Simon, and Michel Boivin. 1998. "Attachment to Parents, Social Support Expectations, and Socioemotional Adjustment during the High School–College Transition." *Journal of Research on Adolescence* 8(1):1–27.

Larose, S., F. Guay, and M. Boivin. 2002. "Attachment, Social Support, and Loneliness in Young Adulthood: A Test of Two Models." *Personality and Social Psychology Bulletin* 28(5):684–693.

Larson, Justine J., Sarah W. Whitton, Stuart T. Hauser, and Joseph P. Allen. 2007. "Being Close and Being Social: Peer Ratings of Distinct Aspects of Young Adult Social Competence." *Journal of Personality Assessment* 89(2):136–148.

Larson, Reed, and Maryse H. Richards. 1991. "Daily Companionship in Late Childhood and Early Adolescence: Changing Development Contexts." *Child Development* 62:284–300.

Larson, Reed W. 2000. "Toward a Psychology of Positive Youth Development." *American Psychologist* 55(1):170–183.

Lauglo, Jon. 2011. "Political Socialization in the Family and Young People's Educational Achievement and Ambition." *British Journal of Sociology of Education* 32(1):53–74.

Lavy, Shiri, Mario Mikulincer, and Phillip R. Shaver. 2010. "Autonomy's Proximity Imbalance: An Attachment Theory Perspective on Intrusiveness in Romantic Relationships." *Personality & Individual Differences* 48:552–556.

Law, K. M., Z. M. Zhang, and S. S. Leung. 2000. "Clothing Deprivation, Clothing Satisfaction, Fashion Leadership and Hong Kong Young Consumers." *Journal of Fashion Marketing & Management* 4:289–302.

Lawrence, Rod. 2000. "Education in China: Preparation for Citizenship." *Asian Affairs* 31(3):273–284.

Lee, Alice Y. L., and Ka Wan Ting. 2015. "Media and Information Praxis of Young Activists in the Umbrella Movement." *Chinese Journal of Communication* 8(4):376–392.

Lee, Francis L. F., Hsuan-Ting Chen, and Michael Chan. 2017. "Social Media Use and University Students' Participation in a Large-Scale Protest Campaign: The Case of Hong Kong's Umbrella Movement." *Telematics & Informatics* 34(2):457–469.

Lee, Kaman. 2009. "Gender Differences in Hong Kong Adolescent Consumers' Green Purchasing Behavior." *Journal of Consumer Marketing* 26(2):87–96.

Lee, Mingun, and Anne E. Fortune. 2013. "Do We Need More Doing Activities or Thinking Activities in the Field Practicum?" *Journal of Social Work Education* 49:646–660.

Lee, Wing On, and Chi Hang Ho. 2005. "Ideological Shifts and Changes in Moral Education Policy in China." *Journal of Moral Education* 34(4):413–431.

LeMare, Lucy J., and Kenneth H. Rubin. 1987. "Perspective Taking and Peer Interaction: Structural and Developmental Analysis." *Child Development* 58:306–315.

Lempers, Jacques D., and Dania S. Clark-Lempers. 1993. "Functional Comparison of Same-sex and Opposite-sex Friendships during Adolescence." *Journal of Adolescent Research* 8(1):89–108.

Leonard, P. 1984. *Personality and Ideology: Towards a Materialist Understanding of the Individual*. London: Macmillan Press.

Lerner, R. M., and C. K. Olson. 1995. "Teen Idols." *Parents* 70:91–92.

Lessard, Jared, Ellen Greenberger, Chuansheng Chen, and Susan Farruggia. 2011. "Are Youths' Feelings of Entitlement Always Bad? Evidence for a Distraction between

Exploitive and Non-exploitive Dimensions of Entitlement." *Journal of Adolescence* 34:521–529.

Leung, L. K. 1999. *Study on the Influence of Media on Youth.* Commission on Youth, Hong Kong Government. Hong Kong, China: Hong Kong Government.

Lever, Joaquina Palomar, Nuria Lanzagorta Pinol, and Jorge Hernandez Uralde. 2005. "Poverty, Psychological Resources and Subjective Well-being." *Social Indicators Research* 73:375–408.

Levpuscek, Melita Puklek, and Maja Zupancic. 2009. "Math Achievement in Early Adolescence: The Role of Parental Involvement, Teachers' Behavior, and Students' Motivational Beliefs about Math." *Journal of Early Adolescence* 29(4):541–570.

Levy, E. 1990. "Social Attributes of American Movie Stars." *Media, Culture & Society* 12(2):247–267.

Lew, Angela S., Rhianon Allen, Nicholas Papouchis, and Barry Ritzler. 1998. "Achievement Orientations and Fear of Success in Asian American College Students." *Journal of Clinical Psychology* 54(1):97–108.

Leybman, Michelle J., David C. Zuroff, Marc A. Fournier, Allison C. Kelly, and Martin Alia. 2011. "Social Exchange Styles: Measurement, Validation, and Application." *European Journal of Personality* 25(3):198–210.

Liang, Belle, Allison Tracy, Maureen Kenny, and Deirdre Brogan. 2008. "Gender Differences in the Relational Health of Youth Participating in a Social Competency Program." *Journal of Community Psychology* 36(4):499–514.

Liao, Minli, Alvin Shiulain Lee, Amelia C. Roberts-Lewis, Jun Sung Hong, and Kaishan Jiao. 2011. "Child Maltreatment in China: An Ecological Review of the Literature." *Children and Youth Services Review* 33(9):1709–1719.

Lichtenstein, Gregg A. 1999. "Building Social Capital: A New Strategy for retaining and Revitalizing Inner-city Manufacturers." *Economic Development Commentary* 23(3):31–38.

Liebler, Carolyn A., and Gary D. Sandefur. 2002. "Gender Differences in the Exchange of Social Support with Friends, Neighbors, and Coworkers at Midlife." *Social Science Research* 31:364–391.

Light, John M., Joel W. Grube, Patricia A. Madden, and Jill Gover. 2003. "Adolescent Alcohol Use and Suicidal Ideation: A Nonrecursive Model." *Addictive Behaviors* 28:705–724.

Light, M. John, and Thomas J. Dishion. 2007. "Early Adolescent Antisocial Behavior and Peer Rejection: A Dynamic Test of a Developmental Process." *New Directions for Child & Adolescent Development* 118:77–89.

Lim, Tock Keng. 1995. "Perceptions of Classroom Environment School Type, Gender and Learning Styles of Secondary School Students." *Educational Psychology* 15(2):161–169.

Lin, Ying-ching, and Chien-Hsin Lin. 2007. "Impetus for Worship: An Exploratory Study of Adolescents' Idol Adoration Behaviors." *Adolescence* 42(167):575–588.

Lindenberg, Siegwart, Janneke F. Joly, and Diederik A. Stapel. 2011. "The Norm-Activating Power of Celebrity: The Dynamics of Success and Influence." *Social Psychology Quarterly* 74(1):98–120.

Lindenmeier, Jorg. 2008. "Promoting Volunteerism: Effects of Self-efficacy, advertisement-induced Emotional Arousal, Perceived Cost of Volunteering, and Message Framing." *Voluntas* 19:43–65.

Liu, Chenying, Tsunetsugu, Munakata, and Francis N. Onuoha. 2005. "Mental Health Condition of the Only-child: A Study of Urban and Rural High School Students in China." *Adolescence* 40(160):831–845.

Liu, Ou Lydia, Frank Rijmen, Carolyn MacCann, and Richard Roberts. 2009. "The Assessment of Time Management in Middle-school Students." *Personality & Individual Differences* 47:174–179.

Liu, Ruth X., Wei Lin, and Zeng-yin Chen. 2010. "School Performance, Peer Association, Psychological and Behavioral Adjustment: A Comparison between Chinese Adolescents with and without Siblings." *Journal of Adolescence* 33:411–417.

Liu, Zhengjia, and Dan Berkowitz. 2014. "Where Is Our Steve Jobs? A Case Study of Consumerism and Neo-Liberal Media in China." *Journalism* 15(8):1006–1022.

Livingstone, Sonia, Nick Couldry, and Tim Markham. 2007. "Youthful Steps towards Civic Participation: Does the Internet Help?" pp. 21–34 in *Young Citizens in the Digital Age: Political Engagement, Young People and New Media*, edited by Brian D. Loader. London: Routledge.

Lopez, Frederick G., and Barbara Gormley. 2002. "Stability and Change in Adult Attachment Style Over the First-Year College Transition: Relations to Self-Confidence, Coping, and Distress Patterns." *Journal of Counseling Psychology* 49(3):355–364.

Lopez, Frederick G., Katherine Ramos, Max Nisenbaum, Navneet Thind, and Tierra Ortiz-Rodriguez. 2014. "Predicting the Presence and Search for Life Meaning: Test of an Attachment Theory-driven Model." *Journal of Happiness Studies* 16:103–116.

Lorant, Vincent, and Pablo Nicaise. 2015. "Binge Drinking at University: A Social Network Study in Belgium." *Health Promotion International* 30(3):675–683.

Lowe, Graham S., and Harvey Krahn. 2000. "Work Aspirations and Attitudes in an Era of Labour Market Restructuring: A Comparison of Two Canadian Youth Cohorts." *Work, Employment and Society* 14(1):1–22.

Lowndes, Vivien, and Mark Roberts. 2013. *Why Institutions Matter: The New Institutionalism in Political Science*. Houndmills, UK: Palgrave.

Lucas, Kristen, and John L. Sherry. 2004. "Sex Difference in Video Game Play: A Communication-based Explanation." *Communication Research* 31(5):499–523.

Luk, Pattie Yuk Yee Fong. 2001. "Comparing Contexts for Developing Personal and Social Education in Hong Kong." *Comparative Education* 37(1):65–87.

Lull, J. 1987. "Listeners' Communicative Uses of Popular Music." pp. 140–174 in *Popular Music and Communication*, edited by J. Lull. Newbury Park, CA: Sage.

Lusardi, Annamaria, Olivia S. Mitchell, and Vilsa Curto. 2010. "Financial Literacy among the Young." *Journal of Consumer Affairs* 44(2):358–380.

Lussier, Gretchen, Kirby Deater-Deckard, Judy Dunn, and Lisa Davies. 2002. "Support across Two Generations: Children's Closeness to Grandparents Following Parental Divorce and Remarriage." *Journal of Family Psychology* 16(3):363–376.

Luszczynska, Aleksandra, and Benicio Gutierrez-Dona. 2005. "General Self-efficacy in Various Domains of Human Functioning: Evidence from Five Countries." *International Journal of Psychology* 40(2):80–89.

Lyubomirsky, S., and H. S. Lepper. 1999. "A Measure of Subjective Happiness: Preliminary Reliability and Construct Validation." *Social Indicators Research* 46(2):137–155.

Ma, Ngok. 2011b. "Value Changes and Legitimacy Crisis in Post-industrial Hong Kong." *Asian Survey* 51(4):683–712.

MacPhee, D., J. C. Kreutzer, and J. J. Pritz. 1994. "Infusing a Diversity Perspective into Human Development Courses." *Child Development* 65:699–715.

Madhavan, Sangeetha, and Jacqueline Crowell. 2014. "Who Would You Like to Be Like? Family, Village, and National Role Models among Black Youth in Rural South Africa." *Journal of Adolescent Research* 29(6):716–737.

Maltby, J. 1999. "The Internal Structure of a Derived, Revised, and Amended Measure of the Religious Orientation Scale: The 'Age-Universal' I-E Scale-12." *Social Behavior and Personality* 27(4):407–412.

Maltby, J. R., M. T. Beriault, N. C. Watson, D. J. Liepert, and G. H. Fick. 2003. "LMA-Classic™ and LMA-ProSeal™ Are Effective Alternatives to Endotracheal Intubation for Gynecologic Laparoscopy." *Canadian Journal of Anesthesia* 50(1):71–77.

Maltby, J., and L. Day. 2001. "The Relationship between Spirituality and Eysenck's Personality Dimensions: A Replication among English Adults." *The Journal of Genetic Psychology* 162(1):119–122.

Maltby, John, Liz Day, David Giles, Raphael Gillett, Marianne Quick, Honey Langcaster-James, and P. Alex Linley. 2008. "Implicit Theories of a Desire for Fame." *British Journal of Psychology* 99(2):279–292.

Maltby, J., L. Day, L. E. McCutcheon, J. Houran, and D. Ashe. 2006. "Extreme Celebrity Worship, Fantasy Proneness and Dissociation: Developing the Measurement and Understanding of Celebrity Worship within a Clinical Personality Context." *Personality and Individual Differences* 40(2):273–283.

Maltby, J., L. Day, L. E. McCutcheon, M. M. Martin, and J. L. Cayanus. 2004. "Celebrity Worship: Cognitive Flexibility, and Social Complexity." *Personality and Individual Differences* 37:1475–1482.

Maltby, J., D. C. Giles, L. Barber, and L. E. McCutcheon. 2005. "Intense-Personal Celebrity Worship and Body Image: Evidence of a Link among Female Adolescents." *British Journal of Health Psychology* 10:17–32.

Maltby, J., J. Houran, L. E. McCutcheon. 2003. "Locating Celebrity Worship within Eysenck's Personality Dimensions." *Journal of Nervous and Mental Disease* 191:25–29.

Maltby, J., J. Houran, R. Lange, D. Ashe, and L. E. McCutcheon. 2002. "Thou Shalt Worship No Other Gods—Unless They Are Celebrities: The Relationship between Celebrity Worship and Religious Orientation." *Personality and Individual Differences* 32(7):1157–1172.

Maltby, J., L. E. McCutcheon, and R. J. Lowinger. 2011. "Brief Report: Celebrity Worshipers and the Five-factor Model of Personality." *North American Journal of Psychology* 13(2):343–348.

Maltby, J., L. E. McCutcheon, D. D. Ashe, and J. Houran. 2001. "The Self-reported Psychological Well-being of Celebrity Worshippers." *North American Journal of Psychology* 3(3):441.

Maltby, John, Liza Day, Lynn E. Mccutcheon, Raphael Gillett, James Houran, and Diane D. Ashe. 2004a. "Personality and Coping: A Context for Examining Celebrity Worship and Mental Health." *British Journal of Psychology* 95:411–428.

Man, T. H. 2013. "Idol Worship, Religiosity and Mental Well-being: A Study of Adolescents in Hong Kong." Undergraduate Thesis, City University of Hong Kong.

Mandell, Lewis, and Linda Schmid Klein. 2009. "The Impact of Financial Literacy Education on Subsequent Financial Behavior." *Journal of Financial Counseling & Planning* 20(1):15–24.

Marazyan, Karine. 2011. "Effects of a Sibship Extension to Father Children on Children's School Environment: A Sibling Rivalry Analysis for Indonesia." *Journal of Development Studies* 47(3):497–518.

Marcia, J. E. 1980. "Identity in Adolescence." pp. 159–187 in *Handbook of Adolescent Psychology*, edited by J. Adelson. New York: John Wiley & Sons.

Marcia, J. E. 1993. "The Ego Identity Status Approach to Ego Identity." pp. 101–121 in *Ego Identity: A Handbook for Psychosocial Research*, edited by J. Marcia, A. Waterman, D. Matteson, SL Archer, and L. Orlofsky. New York, NY: Springer-Verlag.

Marcos, Anastasios C., and Stephen J. Bahr. 1988. "Control Theory and Adolescent Drug Use." *Youth & Society* 19(4):395–425.

Marcotte, Melissa A. 2016. "Individual Differences in Interpretations of Justified and Unjustified Violence." *Peace & Conflict: Journal of Peace Psychology* 22(4):393–395.

Markiewicz, Dorothy, Anna Beth Doyle, and Mara Brendgen. 2001. "The Quality of Adolescents' Friendships: Associations with Mothers' Interpersonal Relationships, Attachments to Parents and Friends, and Prosocial Behaviors." *Journal of Adolescence* 24(4):429–445.

Markoulis, Diomedes, and Nikolaos Valanides. 1997. "Antecedent Variables for Sociomoral Reasoning Development: Evidence from Two Cultural Settings." *International Journal of Psychology* 32(5):301–313.

Marks, Helen M., and Susan Robb Jones. 2004. "Community Service in the Transition: Shifts and Continuities in Participation for High School to College." *Journal of Higher Education* 75(2):307–339.

Marks, Gary N. 2005. "Issues in the School-to-work Transition: Evidence from the Longitudinal Surreys of Australia Youth." *Journal of Sociology* 41(4):363–383.

Markstrom, Carol A., Sheila K. Marshall, and Robin J. Tryon. 2000. "Resiliency, Social Support, and Coping in Rural Low-Income Appalachian Adolescents from Two Racial Groups." *Journal of Adolescence* 23(6):693–703.

Marsh, H. W., K. T. Hau, and Z. Wen. 2004. "In Search of Golden Rules: Comment on Hypothesis-Testing Approaches to Setting Cutoff Values for Fit Indexes and Dangers in Overgeneralizing Hu and Bentler's (1999) Findings." *Structural Equation Modeling* 11:320–341.

Martin, L., and K. Segrave. 1988. *Anti-rock: The Opposition to Rock'n'roll*. Hamden, Conn.: Archon Books.

Martin, Nathan D. 2009. "Social Capital, Academic Achievement, and Postgraduation Plans at an Elite, Private University." *Sociological Perspectives* 52(2):185–210.

Martin, Rod A. 2007. *The Psychology of Humor: An Integrative Approach*. Burlington, MA: Elsevier.

Marzana, Daniela, Elena Marta, Maura Pozzi. 2012. "Social Action in Young Adults: Voluntary and Political Engagement." *Journal of Adolescence* 35:497–507.

Matthews, Todd L., and Frank M. Howell. 2006. "Promoting Civic Culture: The Transmission of Civic Involvement from Parent to Child." *Sociological Focus* 39(1):19–35.

Mayet, Aurelie, Stephane Legleye, Bruno Falissard, and Nearkasen Cahu. 2012. "Cannabis Use Stages as Predictors of Subsequent Initiation with Other Illicit Drugs among French Adolescents: Use of a Multi-state Model." *Addictive Behaviors* 37:160–166.

McCarthy, Bill, and Teresa Casey. 2008. "Love, Sex, and Crime Adolescent Romantic Relationships and Offending." *American Sociological Review* 73:944–969.

McCarthy, Bill, Diane Felmlee, and John Hagan. 2004. "Friends Are Better: Gender, Friends, and Crime among School and Street Youth." *Criminology* 42:805–835.

McCormick, C. B., and J. H. Kennedy. 1994. Parent-child Attachment Working Models and Self-esteem in Adolescence." *Journal of Youth and Adolescence* 23(1):1–18.

McCutcheon, Lynn E., Rense Lange, and James Houran. 2002. "Conceptualization and Measurement of Celebrity Worship." *British Journal of Psychology* 93(1):67–87.

McCutcheon, Lynn E., Diane D. Ashe, James Houran, and John Maltby. 2003. "A Cognitive Profile of Individuals Who Tend to Worship Celebrities." *Journal of Psychology* 137(4):309–322.

McCutcheon, L. E., M. Aruguete, V. B. Scott, and K. L. Von Waldner. 2004. "Preference for Solitude and Attitude towards One's Favorite Celebrity." *North American Journal of Psychology* 6(3):499–506.

McCutcheon, L. E., V. B. Scott Jr., M. S. Aruguete, and J. Parker. 2006. "Exploring the Link between Attachment and the Inclination to Obsess about or Stalk Celebrities." *North American Journal of Psychology* 8(2):289–300.

McElbaney, Kathleen Boykin, Joseph P. Allen, J. Claire Stephenson, and Amanda L. Hare. 2009. "Attachment and Autonomy during Adolescence." pp. 358–463 in *Handbook of Adolescent Psychology, Vol.1: Individual Bases of Adolescent Development*, edited by Richard M. Lerner and Laurence Steinberg. Hoboken, NJ: Wiley.

McEwen, Beryl C. 1994. "Teaching Critical Thinking Skills in Business Education." *Journal of Education for Business* 70(2):99–103.

McLellan, Jeffrey A., and James Youniss. 2003. "Two Systems of Youth Service: Determinants of Voluntary and Required Youth's Community Service." *Journal of Youth & Adolescence* 32(1):47–58.

McMahon, Sarah, N. Andrew Peterson, Samantha C. Winter, Jane E. Palmer, Judy L. Postmus, and Ruth Anne Koenick. 2015. "Predicting Bystander Behavior to Prevent Sexual Assault on College Campuses: The Role of Self-Efficacy and Intent." *American Journal of Community Psychology* 56(1–2):46–56.

McWhirter, Ellen Hawley. 1994. *Counseling for Empowerment*. Alexandra, VA: American Counseling Association.

Meeus, Wim, Annereke, Oosterwegel, and Wilma Vollebergh. 2002. "Parental and Peer Attachment and Identity Development in Adolescence." *Journal of Adolescence* 25:93–106.

Meier, Ann, and Gina Allen. 2008. "Intimate Relationship Development during Transition to Adulthood: Differences by Social Class." *New Directions for Child & Adolescent Development* 119:25–39.

Meloy, J. R. (Ed.). 1998. "The Psychology of Stalking: Clinical and Forensic Perspectives." San Diego, CA: Academic Press.

Melton, H. C. 2000. "Stalking: A Review of the Literature and Direction for the Future." *Criminal Justice Review* 25(2):246–262.

Mesch, Gustavo. 2001. "Social Relationships and Internet Use among Adolescents in Israel." *Social Science Quarterly* 82(2):329–339.

Mikulincer, M. 1995. "Attachment Style and the Mental Representation of the Self." *Journal of Personality and Social Psychology* 69(6):1203.

Mikulincer, M. 1998. "Attachment Working Models and the Sense of Trust: An Exploration of Interaction Goals and Affect Regulation." *Journal of Personality and Social Psychology* 74(5):1209.

Mikulincer, Mario, and Michal Selinger. 2001. "The Interplay between Attachment and Affiliation Systems in Adolescents' Same-Sex Friendships: The Role of Attachment Style." *Journal of Social & Personal Relationships* 18(1):81–106.

Milioni, Michela, Guido Alessandri, Nancy Eisenberg, Valeria Castellani, Antonio Zuffianò, Michele Vecchione, and Gian Vittorio Caprara. 2015. "Reciprocal Relations between Emotional Self-Efficacy Beliefs and Ego-Resiliency across Time." *Journal of Personality* 83(5):552–563.

Miller, Brent C., J. Kelly McCoy, Terrance D. Olson, and Christopher M. Wallace. 1986. "Parental Discipline and Control Attempts in Relation to Adolescent Sexual Attitudes and Behavior." *Journal of Marriage and the Family* 48:503–512.

Miller, Judi Beinstein, and Tvva Hoicoisitz. 2004. "Attachment Context of Adolescent Friendship and Romance." *Journal of Adolescence* 27:191–206.

Millings, Abigail, Rhiannon Buck, Alan Montgomery, Melissa Spears, and Paul Stallard. 2012. "School Connectedness, Peer Attachment, and Self-Esteem as Predictors of Adolescent Depression." *Journal of Adolescence* 35(4):1061–1067.

Miner, M. 2009. "The Impact of Child-Parent Attachment, Attachment to God and Religious Orientation on Psychological Adjustment." *Journal of Psychology and Theology* 37(2):114–124.

Misra, Joya. 1997. "Teaching Stratification: Stimulating Interest and Critical Thinking through Research Projects." *Teaching Sociology* 25:278–291.

Mohr, Jonathan, Rachel Cook-Lyon, and Misty R. Kolchakian. 2010. "Love Imagined: Working Models of Future Romantic Attachment in Emerging Adults." *Personal Relationships* 17(3):457–473.

Monahan, Kathryn C., Laurence Steinberg, Elizabeth Cauffman, and Edward P. Mulvey. 2013. "Psychosocial (Im)maturity from Adolescence to Early Adulthood: Distinguishing between Adolescence-limited and Persisting Antisocial Behavior." *Development & Psychopathology* 25(4):1093–1105.

Moneta, Giovanni B., Barbara Schneider, and Mihaly Csikszentmihalyi. 2001. "A Longitudinal Study of the Self-concept and Experiential Components of Self-worth and Affect across Adolescence." *Applied Developmental Science* 5(2):125–142.

Monteoliva, Adelaida, J. Miguel A. Garcia-Martinez, and Antonia Calvo-Salguero. 2016. "Perceived Benefits and Costs of Romantic Relationships for Young People: Differences by Adult Attachment Style." *Journal of Psychology* 150(8):931–948.

Montepase, Joann M., and Leslie A. Zebrowitz. 2002. "A Social-developmental View of Ageism." pp. 77–125 in *Stereotyping and Prejudice against Older Persons*, edited by Todd D. Nelson. Cambridge, MA: MIT Press.

Moody, James, and Douglas R. White. 2003. "Structural Cohesion and Embeddedness: A Hierarchical Concept of Social Groups." *American Sociological Review* 68:103–127.

Mooney, Karen S., Brett Laursen, and Ryan E. Adams. 2007. "Social Support and Positive Development: Looking on the Bright Side of Adolescent Close Relationships." pp. 189–203 in *Approaches to Positive Youth Development*, edited by Rainer K. Sibereisen and Richard M. Lerner. London: Sage.

Moore, Helen, and Bruce Keith. 1992. "Human Capital and Integration and Tournaments: A Test of Graduate Student Success Models." *American Sociologist* 23(2):52–71.

Morgan, Elizabeth M., and Neill Korobov. 2012. "Interpersonal Identity Formation in Conversations with Close Friends about Dating Relationships." *Journal of Adolescence* 35(6):1471–1483.

Morgan, Stephen L., and Aage B. Sorensen. 1999. "Parental Networks, Social Closure, and Mathematics Learning: A Test of Coleman's Social Capital Explanation of School Effects." *American Sociological Review* 64(5):661–681.

Moriarty, Anthony. 1992. *The Psychology of Adolescent Satanism: A Guide for Parents, Counselors, Clergy, and Teachers*. Westport, CT: Praeger.

Morrison, Elizabeth Wolfe, Ya-ru Chen, and Susan Reilly Salgado. 2004. "Cultural Differences in Newcomer Feedback Seeking: A Comparison of the United States and Hong Kong." *Applied Psychology* 53(1):1–22.

Mortimer, Jeylan T. 2003. *Working and Growing up in America*. Cambridge, MA: Harvard.

Mortimer, Jeylan T., Jeremy Staff, and Sabrina Desterle. 2003. "Adolescent Work and the Early Socioeconomic Career." pp. 437–459 in *Handbook of the Life Course*, edited by Jeylan T. Mortimer and Michael J. Shanahan. New York: Kluwer.

Moseley, Christine, and Juliana Utley. 2008. "An Exploratory Study of Preservice Teachers' Beliefs about the Environment." *Journal of Environmental Education* 39(4):15–29.

Mulder, Clara H., and Michael Wagner. 1998. "First-time Home-ownership in the Family Life Course: A West German-Dutch Comparison." *Urban Studies* 35(4):687–713.

Mulroy, Elizabeth A. 1997. "Building a Neighborhood Network: Interorganizational Collaboration to Prevent Child Abuse and Neglect." *Social Work* 42(3):255–263.

Munch, Richard. 1987. *Theory of Action: Towards a New Synthesis Going beyond Parsons*. London: Routledge & Kegan Paul.

Naftali, Orna. 2009. "Empowering the Child: Children's Rights, Citizenship and the State in Contemporary China. *China Journal* 61:79–103.

Nee, Victor. 2005. "The New Institutionalisms in Economics and Sociology." pp. 49–74 in *The Handbook of Economic Sociology*, 2nd ed, edited by Neil J. Smelser and Richard Swedberg. Princeton, NJ: Princeton University Press.

Nelson, Larry J., and Carolyn McNamara Barry. 2005. "Distinguishing Features of Emerging Adulthood: The Role of Self-Classification as an Adult." *Journal of Adolescent Research* 20(2):242–262.

Newman, Barbara M., Brenda J. Lohman, and Philip R. Newman. 2007. "Peer Group Membership and Sense of Belonging: Their Relationship to Adolescent Behavior Problems." *Adolescence* 42(166):241–263.

Ng, Hoi-Yu. 2015. "Pathways into Political Party Membership: Case Studies of Hong Kong Youth." *Qualitative Report* 20(9):1527–1545.

Niehuis, Sylvia. 2006. "Organization of Partner Knowledge, Its Effect on Passion, and the Mediating Effect of Idealization." *North American Journal of Psychology* 8(1):33–45.\105–305

Niemi, Richard G., Mary A. Hepburn, and Chris Chapman. 2000. "Community Service by High School Student? A Cure for Civic Ills?" *Political Behavior* 22(1):45–69.

Niemi, Richard G., and Jonathan D. Klingler. 2012. "The Development of Political Attitudes and Behaviour among Young Adults." *Australian Journal of Political Science* 47(1):31–54.

Nishikawa, Saori, Elisabet Sundbom, and Bruno Hagglof. 2010. "Influence of Perceived Parental Rearing on Adolescent Self-concepts and Internalizing and Externalizing Problems in Japan." *Journal of Child & Family Studies* 19:57–66.

Niu, Han-Jen, and Yau-de Wang. 2009. "Work Experience Effect on Idolatry and the Impulsive Buying Tendencies of Adolescents." *Adolescence* 44(173):233–243.

North, Adiran C., Lucy Desborough, and Line Skarstein. 2005. "Musical Preference, Deviance, and Attitudes towards Music Celebrities." *Personality & Individual Differences* 38:1903–1914.

Noser, Amy, and Virgil Zeigler-Hill. 2014. "Self-Esteem Instability and the Desire for Fame." *Self and Identity* 13(6):701–713.

Nosko, Amanda, Thanh-Thanh Tieu, Heather Lawford, and Michael W. Pratt. 2011. "How Do I Love Thee? Let Me Count The Ways: Parenting during Adolescence, Attachment Styles, and Romantic Narratives in Emerging Adulthood." *Developmental Psychology* 47(3):645–657.

Nucci, Larry. 2006. "Education for Moral Development." pp. 657–681 in *Handbook of Moral Development*, edited by Melanie Killen and Judith S. Smetana. Mahwah, NJ: Lawrence Erlbaum.

O'Boyle, Edward J. 2005. "Homo Socio-economics: Foundational to Social Economics and the Social Economy." *Review of Social Economy* 63(3):483–507.

O'Connor, Pat, Amanda Haynes, and Ciara Kane. 2004. "Relational Discourses: Social Ties with Family and Friends." *Childhood* 11(3):361–382.

O'Koon, J. 1997. "Attachment to Parents and Peers in Late Adolescence and Their Relationship with Self-image." *Adolescence* 32(126):471.

Oksanen, Atte, James Hawdon, Emma Holkeri, Matti Näsi, Pekka Räsänen, and M. Nicole Warehime. 2014. "Exposure to Online Hate among Young Social Media Users." *Sociological Studies of Children & Youth* 18:267–273.

Oldmeadow, Julian, and Susan T. Fiske. 2007. "System-justifying Ideologies Moderate Status = Competence Stereotypes: Roles for Belief in a Just World and Social Dominance Orientation." *European Journal of Social Psychology* 37:1135–1148.

Onu, Diana, Thomas Kessler, Daniela Andonovska-Trajkovska, Immo Fritsche, Georgia R. Midson, and Joanne R. Smith. 2016. "Inspired by the Outgroup: A Social Identity Analysis of Intergroup Admiration." *Group Processes & Intergroup Relations* 19(6):713–731.

Ooi, Y. P., R. P. Ang, D. S. Fung, G. Wong, and Y. Cai, 2006. "The Impact of Parent-child Attachment on Aggression, Social Stress and Self-esteem." *School Psychology International* 27(5):552–566.

Ovadia, Seth. 2001. "Race, Class, and Gender Differences in High School Seniors' Values: Applying Intersection Theory in Empirical Analysis." *Social Science Quarterly* 82(2):340–356.

Owens, Laurence, Anthony Daly, and Phillip Slee. 2005. "Sex and Age Differences in Victimisation and Conflict Resolution among Adolescents in a South Australian School." *Aggressive Behavior* 31:1–12.

Parade, Stephnie H., Esther M. Leekes, and A. Nayena Blankson. 2010. "Attachment to Parents, Social Anxiety, and Close Relationships of Female Students over the Transition to College." *Journal of Youth & Adolescence* 39:127–137.

Pargament, K. I. 1997. *The Psychology of Religion and Coping: Theory, Research, Practice.* New York: Guilford Press.

Parks, Acacia C., Stephen M. Schueller, and Arber Tasimi. 2014. "Increasing Happiness in the General Population: Empirically Supported Self-help?" pp. 962–977 in the *Oxford Handbook of Happiness,* edited by Susan A. David, Ilona Boniwell, and Amanda Conley Ayers. Oxford, UK: Oxford University Press.

Parsons, Talcott. 1968. *The Structure of Social Action.* New York: Free Press.

Patall, Erika A., Harris Cooper, and Jorgianne Civey Robinson. 2008. "The Effects of Choice of Intrinsic Motivation and Related Outcomes: A Meta-analysis of Research Findings." *Psychological Bulletin* 134(2):270–300.

Paterson, J., J. Pryor, and J. Field. 1995. "Adolescent Attachment to Parents and Friends in Relation to Aspects of Self-esteem." *Journal of Youth and Adolescence* 24(3):365–376.

Pattie, Charles, Patrick Seyd, and Paul Whiteley. 2004. *Citizenship in Britain: Values, Participation and Democracy.* Cambridge, UK: Cambridge University Press.

Pellegrini, Anthony D., and Peter Blatchford. 2000. *The Child at School: Interactions with Peers and Teachers.* London: Arnold.

Peltonen, Kirsi, Samir Quota, Eyad Elsarraj, and Raija-Leena Punamaki. 2010. "Military Trauma and Social Development: The Moderating and Mediating Roles of Peer and Sibling Relations in Mental Health." *International Journal of Behavioral Development* 34:554–563.

Peng, Jin, Jianbo Shao, Huiping Zhu, Chuanhua Yu, Wenyan Yao, Hongyan Yao, Junxin Shi, and Huiyun Xian. 2015. "A Systems Approach to Addressing Child Maltreatment in China: China Needs a Formalized Child Protection System." *Child Abuse & Neglect* 50:33–41.

Peng, Kaiping, and Richard E. Nisbett. 1999. "Culture, Dialectics, and Reasoning about Contradiction." *American Psychologist* 54(9):741–754.

Peng, Wen-bo, Xiao-ting Qiu, Dian-zhi Liu, and Pang Wang. 2010. "Revision of the Scale of Celebrity Worship." *Psychological Development & Education* 2010(5):543–548.

Permuy, Beatriz, Hipólito Merino, and Jose Fernandez-Rey. 2010. "Adult Attachment Styles and Cognitive Vulnerability to Depression in a Sample of Undergraduate Students: The Mediational Roles of Sociotropy and Autonomy." *International Journal of Psychology* 45(1):21–27.

Perron, Brian E., and Matthew O. Howard. 2008. "Perceived Risk of Harm and Intentions of Future Inhalant Use among Adolescent Inhalant Users." *Drug & Alcohol Dependence* 97:185–189.

Perse, E. M., and A. M. Rubin. 1990. "Chronic Loneliness and Television Use." *Journal of Broadcasting & Electronic Media* 34(1):37–53."

Peters, B. Guy. 1999. *Institutional Theory in Political Science: The New Institutionalism.* London: Continuum.

Pfeiffer, Jens P., and Martin Pinquart. 2012. "Goal Engagement and Goal Attainment in Adolescents with and without Visual Impairment." *Journal of Adolescence* 35:909–916.

Piko, Bettina F., Noemi Keresztes, and Zsuzsanna F. Pluhar. 2006. "Aggressive Behavior and Psychosocial Health among Children." *Personality & Individual Differences* 40:885–895.

Pinquart, Martin, and Jens P. Pfeiffer. 2013. "Does Visual Impairment Lead to Lower or Higher Levels of Success in Solving Developmental Tasks? A Longitudinal Study." *Journal of Developmental & Physical Disabilities* 25:579–595.

Pinquart, Martin, Rainer K. Silbereisen, and Linda P. Juang. 2004. "Changes in Psychosocial Distress among East German Adolescents Facing German Unification: The Role of Commitment to the Old System and of Self-efficacy Beliefs." *Youth & Society* 36(1):77–101.

Pires, Paulo, and Jennifer M. Jenkins. 2007. "A Growth Curve Analysis of the Joint Influences of Parenting Affect, Child Characteristics and Deviant Peers on Adolescent Illicit Drug Use." *Youth & Adolescence* 36:169–183.

Pithers, R. T., and Rebecca Soden. 2000. "Critical Thinking in Education: A Review." *Educational Research* 42(3):237–249.

Pleiss, Mary K., and John F. Feldhusen. 1995. "Mentors, Role Models, and Heroes in the Lives of Gifted Children." *Educational Psychologists* 30(3):159–169.

Pong, Suet-ling, Jamie Johnston, and Vivien Chen. 2010. "Authoritarian Parenting and Asian Adolescent School Performance: Insights from the US and Taiwan." *International Journal of Behavioral Development* 34(1):62–72.

Porter, B. F. 1988. *Reasons for Living: A Basic Ethics.* New York: Macmillan.

Power, Ann Marie R., and Vladimir T. Khmelkov. 1999. "The Effects of Service Participation on High School Students' Social Responsibility." *Research in Sociology of Education and Socialization* 12:185–210.

Preckel, Franzis, and Matthias Brull. 2010. "The Benefit of Being a Big Fish in a Big Pond: Contrast and Assimilation Effects on Academic Self-concept." *Learning & Individual Differences* 20:522–531.

Price, Jennifer L., Robert J. Lowinger, William Jenkins, and Lynn E. McCutcheon. 2014. "The Stigmatization of People with a History of Mental Illness by Those Who Admire Celebrities." *North American Journal of Psychology* 16(2):253–260.

Prinstein, Mitchell J. 2007. "Moderators of Peer Contagion: A Longitudinal Examination of Depression Socialization between Adolescents and Their Beast Friends." *Journal of Clinical Child & Adolescent Psychology* 36(2):159–170.

Prinstein, Mitchell J., Jessica L. Borelli, Charissa S. L. Cheah, Valerie A. Simon, and Julie Wargo Aikens. 2005. "Adolescent Girls' Interpersonal Vulnerability to Depressive Symptoms: A Longitudinal Examination of Reassurance-seeking and Peer Relationships." *Journal of Abnormal Psychology* 114(4):676–688.

Pullmann, H., and J. Allik. 2000. "The Rosenberg Self-Esteem Scale: Its Dimensionality, Stability and Personality Correlates in Estonian." *Personality and Individual Differences* 28:701–715.

Qi, Wanxue, and Hanwei Tang. 2004. "The Social and Cultural Background of Contemporary Moral Education in China." *Journal of Moral Education* 33(4):465–480.

Quiroga, Manuela Garcia, and Catherine Hamilton-Giachritsis. 2017. "The Crucial Role of the Micro Caregiving Environment: Factors Associated with Attachment Styles in Alternative Care in Chile." *Child Abuse & Neglect* 70:169–179.

Radford, Scott K., and Peter H. Bloch. 2012. "Grief, Commiseration, and Consumption Following the Death of a Celebrity." *Journal of Consumer Culture* 12(2):137–155.

Raja, Shyamala Nada, Rob McGee, and Warren R. Stanton. 1992. "Perceived Attachments to Parents and Peers and Psychological Well-Being in Adolescence." *Journal of Youth and Adolescence* 21(4):471–485.

Rajeev, Dehejia, Thomas DeLeire, Erzo F. P. Luttmer, and Josh Mitchell. 2009. "The Role of Religious and Social Organizations in the Lives of Disadvantaged Youth." pp. 237–274 in *The Problems of Disadvantaged Youth: An Economic Perspective*, edited by Jonathan Gruber. Chicago, IL: University of Chicago Press.

Ramsey, Meagan A., and Amy L. Gentzler. 2015. "An Upward Spiral: Bidirectional Associations between Positive Affect and Positive Aspects of Close Relationships across the Life Span." *Developmental Review* 36:58–104.

Raviv, Amisam, Daniel Bar-Tal, Alona Raviv, and Asaf Ben-Horin. 1996. "Adolescent Idolization of Pop Singers: Causes, Expressions, and Reliance." *Journal of Youth and Adolescence* 25(5):631–650.

Rawlings, Mary A. 2012. "Assessing BSW Student Direct Practice Skill Using Standardized Clients and Self-efficacy Theory." *Journal of Social Work Education* 48(2):553–576.

Read, D., G. R. Adams, and W. R. Dobson. 1984. "Ego-Identity Status, Personality, and Social-Influence Style." *Journal of Personality and Social Psychology* 46(1):169.

Reed, Gay Garland. 1995. "Moral/Political Education in the People's Republic of China: Learning through Role Models." *Journal of Moral Education* 24(2):99–111.

Reed, Jennifer H., and Jeffrey D. Kromrey. 2001. "Teaching Critical Thinking in a Community College History Course: Empirical Evidence from Infusing Paul's Model." *College Student Journal* 35(2):201–215.

Reeves, Robert A., Gary A. Baker, and Chris S. Truluck. 2012. "Celebrity Worship, Materialism Compulsive Buying and the Empty Self." *Psychology & Marketing* 29(9):674–679.

Regnerus, M. D. 2003. "Religion and Positive Adolescent Outcomes: A Review of Research and Theory." *Review of Religious Research* 44:394–413.

Regnerus, Mark D. 2002. "Friends' Influence on Adolescent Theft and Minor Delinquency: A Developmental Test of Peer-reported Effects." *Social Science Research* 31:681–705.

Reijnders, Stijn L., Gerard Rooijakkers, and Liesbet van Zoonen. 2007. "Community Spirit and Competition in Idols: Ritual Meanings of a TV Talent Quest." *European Journal of Communication* 22(3):275–292.

Reio, Thomas G., Robert F. Marcus, and Joanne Sanders-Reio. 2009. "Contribution of Student and Instructor Relationships and Attachment Style to School Completion." *Journal of Genetic Psychology* 170(1):53–72.

Rest, James, Darcia Narvaez, Muriel J. Bebeau, and Stephen J. Thoma. 1999. *Postconventional Moral Thinking: A Neo-Kohlbergian Approach*. Mahwah, NJ: Lawrence Erlbaum.

Reynolds, Andrew D., and Thomas M. Crea. 2015. "Peer Influence Processes for Youth Delinquency and Depression." *Journal of Adolescence* 43:83–95.

Reysen, Stephen, Courtney N. Plante, Sharon E. Roberts, and Kathleen C. Gerbasi. 2016. "Optimal Distinctiveness and Identification with the Furry Fandom." *Current Psychology* 35(4):638–642.

Richardson, George B., Patrick H. Hardesty, and Benjamin Jeppsen. 2015. "Family Idealization Explains the Effect between Family Religiousness and Youth Psychological Functioning." *Journal of Child and Family Studies* 24(5):1243–1255.

Richmond, Aaron S., and Rhoda Cummings. 2004. "In Support of the Cognitive-developmental Approach to Moral Education: A Response to David Carr." *Journal of Moral Education* 33(2):197–205.

Ridenour, Ty A., Mark T. Greenberg, Elizabeth T. Cook. 2006. "Structure and Validity of People in My Life: A Self-report Measure of Attachment in Late Childhood." *Journal of Youth & Adolescence* 35:1037–1053.

Ritzer, George, Douglas Goodman, and Wendy Wiedenhoft. 2001. "Theories of Consumption." pp. 410–427 in *Handbook of Social Theory*, edited by George Ritzer and Barry Smart. London: Sage.

Roberts, Alden E., Jerome R. Koch, and D. Paul Johnson. 2001. "Religious Reference Groups and the Persistence of Normative Behavior: An Empirical Test." *Sociological Spectrum* 21:81–98.

Roberts, James A. 1998. "Compulsive Buying among College Students: An Investigation of Its Antecedents, Consequences, and Implications for Public Policy." *Journal of Consumer Affairs* 32(2):295–319.

Robins, R. W., H. M. Hendin, and K. H. Trzesniewski. 2001. "Measuring Global Self-esteem: Construct Validation of a Single-item Measure and the Rosenberg Self-Esteem Scale." *Personality and Social Psychology Bulletin* 27(2):151–161.

Robinson, Oliver C., Abigail Dunn, Sofya Nartova-Bochaver, Konstantin Bochaver, Samaneh Asadi, Zohreh Khosravi, Seyed Mohammad Jafari, Xiaozhou Zhang, and Yanbo Yang. 2016. "Figures of Admiration in Emerging Adulthood: A Four-Country Study." *Emerging Adulthood* 4(2):82–91.

Roeser, Robert W., Mollie Galloway, Shannon Casey-Cannon, Cary Watson, and Laura Keller, and Elyn Tan. 2008. "Identity Representations in Patterns of School

Achievement and Well-being among Early Adolescent Girls: Variable- and Person-centered Approaches." *Journal of Early Adolescence* 28(1):115–152.

Rogers, Mary E., and Peter A. Creed. 2011. "A Longitudinal Examination of Adolescent Career Planning and Exploration Using a Social Cognitive Career Theory Framework." *Journal of Adolescence* 34(1):163–172.

Rose, Richard J. 2002. "How Do Adolescents Select Their Friends? A Behavior-genetic Perspective." pp. 106–125 in *Paths to Successful Development: Personality in the Life Course*, edited by Lea Pulkkinen and Avshalom Caspi. Cambridge, UK: Cambridge University Press.

Rose-Krasnor, Linda, Michael A. Busseri, Teena Willoughby, and Heather Chalmers. 2005. "Breath and Intensity of Youth Activity Involvement as Contexts of Positive Development." *Journal of Youth & Adolescence* 35(3):385–399.

Rosenberg, Morris. 1965. "Rosenberg Self-Esteem Scale (RSE)." *Acceptance and Commitment Therapy. Measures Package* 61:52.

Rosenfield, Sarah, Mary Clare Lennon, and Helene Raskin White. 2005. "The Self and Mental Health: Self-salience and the Emergence of Internalizing and Externalizing Problems." *Journal of Health & Social Behavior* 46(4):323–340.

Rosenthal, T. L., and B. J. Zimmerman. 1978. "Social Learning and Cognition." New York: Academic Press.

Ross, Catherine E., and John Mirowsky. 1989. "Explaining the Social Patterns of Depression: Control and Problem Solving—or Support and Talking?" *Journal of Health and Social Behavior* 30(2):206–219.

Roth, Guy, and Avi Assor. 2012. "The Costs of Parental Pressure to Express Emotions: Conditional Regard and Autonomy Support as Predictors of Emotion Regulation and Intimacy." *Journal of Adolescence* 35(4):799–808.

Rubin, A. M., E. M. Perse, and R. A. Powell, 1985. "Loneliness, Parasocial Interaction, and Local Television News Viewing." *Human Communication Research* 12(2):155–180.

Rubin, Kenneth, Bridget Fredstrom, and Gulie Bowker. 2008. "Future Directions in Friendship in Childhood and Early Adolescence." *Social Development* 17(4):1085–1096.

Rudasill, K. M., P. Possel, S. Winkeljohn Black, and K. Niehaus. 2014. "Teacher Support Mediates Concurrent and Longitudinal Associations between Temperament and Mild Depressive Symptoms in Sixth Grade." *Early Child Development and Care* 184(6):803–818.

Rusch, Hannes, Joost M. Leunissen, and Markvan Vugt. 2015. "Historical and Experimental Evidence of Sexual Selection for War Heroism." *Evolution & Human Behavior* 36(5):367–373.

Ryu, Sungjin, Susan Kline, and Kim Jinsuk. 2007. "Identification with Television Newscasters and Korean College Students' Voting Intentions and Political Activities." *Asian Journal of Social Psychology* 10(3):188–197.

Salavera, Carlos, Pablo Usán, and Laurane Jarie. 2017. "Emotional Intelligence and Social Skills on Self-Efficacy in Secondary Education Students. Are There Gender Differences?" *Journal of Adolescence* 60:39–46.

Sanchirico, Andrew. 1991. "The Importance of Small-business Ownership in Chinese American Educational Achievement." *Sociology of Education* 64:293–304.

Sanderson, Stephen K. 2001. *The Evolution of Human Sociality: Darwinian Conflict Perspective.* Lanham, MD: Rowman & Littlefield.

Sansone, R. A., and L. A. Sansone. 2014. "I'm Your Number One Fan: A Clinical Look at Celebrity Worship." *Innovations in Clinical Neuroscience* 11(1–2):39–43.

Sarapin, Susan H., Katheryn Christy, Louise Lareau, Melinda Krakow, and Jakob D. Jensen. 2015. "Identifying Admired Models to Increase Emulation: Development of a Multidimensional Admiration Scale." *Measurement & Evaluation in Counseling & Development* 48(2):95–108.

Scales, Peter C., Peter L. Benson, Nancy Leffert, and Dale A. Blyth. 2000. "Contribution of Developmental Assets to the Prediction of Thriving among Adolescents." *Applied Developmental Science* 4(1):27–46.

Scharf, Miri, and Miri Levy. 2015. "The Contribution of Familial Characteristics and Idolization to Children's Body and Eating Attitudes." *Journal of Child & Family Studies* 24(7):1943–1954.

Schee, Carolyn Vander, and Kip Kline. 2013. "Neoliberal Exploitation in Reality Television: Youth, Health and the Spectacle of Celebrity Concern." *Journal of Youth Studies* 16(5):565–578.

Schenke, Katerina, Arena C. Lam, Anne Marie M. Conley, and Stuart A. Karabenick. 2015. "Adolescents' Help Seeking in Mathematics Classrooms: Relations Between Achievement and Perceived Classroom Environmental Influences over One School Year." *Contemporary Educational Psychology* 41:133–146.

Schimmenti, Adriano, and Antonia Bifulco. 2015. "Linking Lack of Care in Childhood to Anxiety Disorders in Emerging Adulthood: The Role of Attachment Styles." *Child & Adolescent Mental Health* 20(1):41–48.

Schindler, Ines, Juliane Paech, and Fabian Lowenbruck. 2015. "Linking Admiration and Adoration to Self-expansion: Different Ways to Enhance One's Potential." *Cognition and Emotion* 29(2):292–310.

Schindler, Ines, Veronika Zink, Johannes Windrich, and Winfried Menninghaus. 2013. "Admiration and Adoration: Their Different Ways of Showing and Shaping Who We Are." *Cognition & Emotion* 27(1):85–118.

Schlenker, Barry R., Michael F. Weigold, and Kristine A. Schlenker. 2008. "What Makes a Hero? The Impact of Integrity on Admiration and Interpersonal Judgment." *Journal of Personality* 76(2):323–355.

Schmitt-Redermund, Eva, and Fred W. Vondracek. 2002. "Occupational Dreams, Choices, and Aspirations: Adolescents' Entrepreneurial Prospect and Orientations." *Journal of Adolescence* 25:65–78.

Schnell, Kerstin, Tobias Ringeisen, Diana Raufelder, Sonja Rohrmann. 2015. "The Impact of Adolescents' Self-Efficacy and Self-Regulated Goal Attainment Processes on School Performance: Do Gender and Test Anxiety Matter?" *Learning & Individual Differences* 38:90–98.

Scholte, Ron H. J., Geertjan Overbeek, Giovanni ten Brink, Els Rommes, Raymond A. T. de Kemp, Luc Goossens, and Rutger G. M. E. Engels. 2009. "The Significance of

Reciprocal and Unilateral Friendships for Peer Victimization in Adolescence." *Journal of Youth & Adolescence* 38:89–100.

Schulenberg, John, Patrick M. O'Malley, Jerald G. Bachman, and Lloyd D. Johnston. 2000. "Spread Your Wings and Fly: The Course of Well-being and Substance Use during the Transition to Young Adulthood." pp. 224–255 in *Negotiating Adolescence in Times of Social Change*, edited by Lisa J. Crockett and Rainer K. Silbereisen. Cambridge, UK: Cambridge University Press.

Schultze, Quentin J., Roy M. Anker, James D. Bratt, William D. Romanowkski, John William Worst, and Lambert Zuidervaart. 1991. *Dancing in the Dark: Youth, Popular Culture, and the Electronic Media*. Grand Rapids, MI: Williams B. Eerdmans.

Schunk, D. H. 1987. "Peer Models and Children's Behavioral Change." *Review of Educational Research* 57(2):149–174.

Schunk, D. H., and A. R. Hanson. 1985. "Peer models: Influence on Children's Self-Efficacy and Achievement." *Journal of Educational Psychology* 77(3):313.

Schunk, Dale H., and Barry J. Zimmerman. 1996. "Modeling and Self-efficacy Influences on Children's Development of Self-regulation." pp. 154–180 in *Social Motivation: Understanding Children's School Adjustment*, edited by Jeana Juvonen, and Kathryn R. Wentzel. Cambridge: Cambridge.

Schutz, Helena K., Susan J. Paxton, and Eleanor H. Wertheim. 2002. "Investigation of Body Comparison among Adolescent Girls." *Journal of Applied Social Psychology* 32(9):1906–1937.

Schwartz, David, Andrea Hopmeyer-Gorman, Robin L. Toblin, and Tania Abau-ezzeddine. 2003. "Mutual Antipathies in the Peer Group as a Moderating Factor in the Association between Community Violence Exposure and Psychosocial Maladjustment." *New Directions for Child & Adolescent Development* 102:39–72.

Schwarzer, Ralf, John Mueller, and Esther Greenglass. 1999. "Assessment of Perceived General Self-Efficacy on the Internet: Data Collection in Cyberspace." *Anxiety, Stress & Coping* 12(2):145–161.

Scott, W. Richard. 2008. *Institutions and Organizations: Ideas and Interests*, 3rd ed. Los Angeles, CA: Sage.

Seibert, Ashley C., and Kathryn A. Kerns. 2009. "Attachment Figures in Middle Childhood." *International Journal of Behavioral Development* 33(4):347–355.

Seiffge-Krenke, Inge. 1997. "Imaginary Companions in Adolescence: Sign of a Deficient or Positive Development?" *Journal of Adolescence* 20(2):137–154.

Shadur, Julia M., and Andrea M. Hussong. 2014. "Friendship Intimacy, Close Friend Drug Use, and Self-Medication in Adolescence." *Journal of Social & Personal Relationships* 31(8):997–1018.

Shamir-Essakow, Galia, Judy A. Ungerer, and Ronald M. Rapee. 2005. "Attachment, Behavioral Inhibition, and Anxiety in Preschool Children." *Journal of Abnormal Child Psychology* 33(2):131–143.

Sharabany, Ruth. 1994. "Intimate Friendship Scale: Conceptual Underpinnings, Psychometric Properties and Construct Validity." *Journal of Social & Personal Relationships* 11(3):449–469.

Shaver, Phillip R., and Mario Mikulincer. 2012. "Attachment Theory." pp. 160–179 in *Handbook of Theories of Social Psychology*, Vol. 2, edited by Paul A. M. Van Lange, Arie W. Kruglanski, and E. Tory Higgins. London, CA: SAGE.

Sheehan, Grania, and Patricia Noller. 2002. "Adolescent's Perceptions of Differential Parenting: Links with Attachment Style and Adolescent Adjustment." *Personal Relationships* 9(2):173–190.

Sheldon, Kennon M., and Holly A. McGregor. 2000. "Extrinsic Value Orientation and the Tragedy of the Commons." *Journal of Personality* 68(2):383–411.

Shen, April Chiang-Too. 2009. "Self-esteem of Young Adults Experiencing Interparental Violence and Child Physical Maltreatment: Parental and Peer Relationships as Mediators." *Journal of Interpersonal Violence* 24(5):770–794.

Shen, J. 2001. "Chinese Youth in 2000." pp. 338–360 in *2000: Analysis and Forecast of China's Social Situation*, edited by L. Jiang, X. Lu, and T. Dan. Beijing, China: China Social Science (in Chinese).

Shepelak, Norma J. 1996. "Employing a Mock Trial in a Criminology Course: An Applied Learning Experience." *Teaching Sociology* 24(4):395–400.

Sheridan, Lorraine, Adrian North, John Maltby, and Raphael Gillett. 2007. "Celebrity Worship, Addiction and Criminality." *Psychology, Crime & Law* 13(6):559–571.

Sheridan, Zachariah, Peter Boman, Amanda Mergler, and Michael J. Furlong. 2015. "Examining Well-being, Anxiety, and Self-deception in University Students." *Cogent Psychology* 2(1):993850.

Sherlock, S. 1997. "The Future of Commodity Fetishism." *Sociological Focus* 30:61–78.

Shimai, Satoshi, Keiko Otake, Nansook Park, Christopher Peterson, and Martin E. P. Seligman. 2006. "Convergence of Character Strengths in American Young Adults." *Journal of Happiness Studies* 7:311–322.

Short, Elizabeth J., Christopher W. Schatschneider, and Sarah E. Friebert. 1992. "The Inactive Learner Hypothesis: Myth or Reality?" pp. 302–326 in *Learning Disabilities: Nature, Theory, and Treatment*, edited by Nirbhay N. Singh and Ivan L. Beale. New York: Springer-Verlag.

Showalter, E. 1997. *Hystories: Hysterial Epidemics and Modern Media*. New York: Columbia University Press.

Simons-Morton, Bruce, and Rusan S. Chen. 2006. "Over Time Relationships between Early Adolescent and Peer Substance Use." *Addictive Behaviors* 31:1211–1223.

Simonton, D. K. 1978. "History and the Eminent Person." *Gifted Child Quarterly* 22:187–195.

Simonton, Dean Keith. 1981. "Formal Education, Eminence, and Dogmatism: The Curvilinear Relationship." *Paper presented at the Annual Meeting of the American Educational Research Association*, Los Angeles, CA: April 13–17.

Simonton, Dean Keith. 1994. *Greatness: Who Makes History and Why*. New York: Guilford.

Singer, M. S., B. G. Stacey, and C. Lange. 1993. "The Relative Utility of Expectancy-value Theory and Social Cognitive Theory in Predicting Psychology Student Course Goals and Career Aspiration." *Journal of Social Behavior and Personality* 8:703–714.

Sivami, Viren, Tomas Chamorro-Premuzic, Khairvl Mastor, Fatin Hazani Siran, Mohammad Mohsein Mohammad Said, Jas Jaafar, Dhachayani Sinniah, and Subash K. Pillas.

2010. "Celebrity Worship among University Students in Malaysia: A Methodological Contribution to the Celebrity Attitude Scale." *European Psychologist* 16(4):334–342.

Sjaastad, Jørgen. 2012. "Sources of Inspiration: The Role of Significant Persons in Young People's Choice of Science in Higher Education." *International Journal of Science Education* 34(10):1615–1636.

Smith, Chris D., and Lindsay Wright. 2000. "Perceptions of Genius: Einstein, Lesser Mortals and Shooting Stars." *Journal of Creative Behavior* 34(3):165–174.

So, C. Y. C., and J. M. Chan. 1992. Mass media and youth in Hong Kong: A study of media use, youth archetype, and media influence. Commission on Youth: Hong Kong Government.

Sobel, Michael E. 1981. *Lifestyle and Social Structure: Concepts, Definitions, Analyses.* New York: Academic Press.

Soenens, Bart, Seong-Yeon Park, Maarten Vansteenkiste, and Athannsios Mouratidis. 2012. "Perceived Parental Psychological Control and Adolescent Depressive Experiences: A Cross-cultural Study with Belgian and South-Korean Adolescents." *Journal of Adolescence* 35:261–272.

Solomon, Robert C. 2003. *Living with Nietzsche: What the Great Immoralist Has to Teach Us.* Oxford, UK: Oxford University Press.

Song, Hairong, Ross A. Thompson, and Emilio Ferrer. 2009. "Attachment and Self-evaluation in Chinese Adolescents: Age and Gender Differences." *Journal of Adolescence* 32:1267–1286.

Southard, Ashton C., and Virgil Zeigler-Hill. 2016. "The Dark Triad Traits and Fame Interest: Do Dark Personalities Desire Stardom?" *Current Psychology* 35(2):255–267.

Sparapani, Erwin F. 1998. "Encouraging Thinking in High School and Middle School: Constraints and Possibilities." *Clearing House* 71(5):274–276.

Spaulding, Sue C., and Kathleen A. Kleiner. 1992. "The Relationship of College and Critical Thinking: Are Critical Thinkers Attracted or Created by College Disciplines?" *College Student Journal* 26(2):162–166.

Spencer-Rodgers, Julie, Melissa J. Williams, and Kaiping Peng. 2010. "Cultural Differences in Expectations of Change and Tolerance for Contradiction: A Decade of Empirical Research." *Personality & Social Psychology Review* 14(3):296–312.

Springer, Kriisten W., Jennifer Sheridan, Daphne Kuo, and Molly Carnes. 2007. "Long-term Physical and Mental Consequences of Childhood Physical Abuse: Results from a Large Population-based Sample of Men and Women." *Child Abuse & Neglect* 31:517–530.

Srivastava, S., and J. S. Beer. 2005. "How Self-evaluations Relate to Being Liked by Others: Integrating Sociometer and Attachment Perspectives." *Journal of Personality and Social Psychology* 89(6):966.

Staff, Jeremy, and Derek A. Kraeger. 2008. "Too Cool for School? Violence, Peer Status and High School Dropout." *Social Forces* 87(1):445–471.

Stanton, Warren R., Greg D. Currie, Tian P.S. Oei, and Phil A. Silva. 1996. "A Developmental Approach to Influences on Adolescents' Smoking and Quitting." *Journal of Applied Developmental Psychology* 17:307–319.

Starrels, Marjorie E., and Kristen E. Holm. 2000. "Adolescents' Plans for Family Formation: Is Parental Socialization Important?" *Journal of Marriage & the Family* 62:416–429.

Steele, Ric G., Jill S. Nesbitt-Daly, Robert C. Daniel, and Rex Forehand. 2005. "Factor Structure of the Parenting Scale in a Low-income African American Sample." *Journal of Child & Family Studies* 14(4):535–549.

Steger, Michael F., and Todd B. Kashdan. 2006. "Stability and Specificity of Meaning in Life and Life Satisfaction over One Year." *Journal of Happiness Studies* 8:161–179.

Stets, Jan E., and Teresa M. Tsushima. 2001. "Negative Emotion and Coping Responses within Identity Control Theory." *Social Psychology Quarterly* 64(3):283–295.

Stevens, Carolyn S. 2010. "You Are What You Buy: Postmodern Consumption and Fandom of Japanese Popular Culture." *Japanese Studies* 30(2):199–214.

Stever, G. 1994. "Para-social Attachments: Motivational Antecedents." *Dissertation Abstracts International* B55/07:3039, January 1995.

Stever, Gayle S. 2008. "The Celebrity Appeal Questionnaire: Sex, Entertainment, or Leadership." *Psychological Reports* 103(1):113–120.

Stever, G. S. 2009. "Parasocial and Social Interaction with Celebrities: Classification of Media Fans." Journal of Media Psychology 14(3):1–39.

Stewart, Charles J., Craig Allen Smith, and Robert E. Denton, Jr. 2012. *Persuasion and Social Movements.* Long Grove, IL: Waveland.

Storvoll, Elisabet, and Lars Wichstrom. 2002. "Do the Risk Factors Associated with Conduct Problems in Adolescents Vary According to Gender?" *Journal of Adolescence* 25:183–202.

Stringer, Kate J., and Jennifer L. Kerpelman. 2010. "Career Identity Development in College Students: Decision Making, Parental Support, and Work Experience." *Identity* 10(3):181–200.

Strohschein, Lisa, and Alvinelle Matthew. 2015. "Adolescent Problem Behavior in Toronto, Canada." *Sociological Inquiry* 85(1):129–147.

Sumter, Sindy R., Patti M. Valkenburg, and Jochen Peter. 2013. "Perceptions of Love across the Lifespan Differences in Passion, Intimacy, and Commitment." *International Journal of Behavioral Development* 37(5):417–427.

Swami, V., T. Chamorro-Premuzic, K. Mastor, F. Hazwani Siran, M. M. M. Said, J. Jaafar, and S. K. Pillai. 2011. "Celebrity Worship among University Students in Malaysia: A Methodological Contribution to the Celebrity Attitude Scale." *European Psychologist* 16(4):334.

Swami, Viren, Rosanne Taylor, and Christine Carvalho. 2009. "Acceptance of Cosmetic Surgery and Celebrity Worship: Evidence of Associations among Female Undergraduates." *Personality & Individual Differences* 47:869–872.

Swank, Eric W. 2012. "Predictors of Political Activism among Social Work Students." *Journal of Social Work Education* 48(2):245–266.

Sweetman, Joseph, Russell Spears, Andrew G. Livingstone, and Antony S. R. Manstead. 2013. "Admiration Regulates Social Hierarchy: Antecedents, Dispositions, and Effects on Intergroup Behavior." *Journal of Experimental Social Psychology* 49(3):534–542.

Szymanski, G. G. 1977. "Celebrities and Heroes as Models of Self-perception." *Journal of the Association for the Study of Perception* 12:8–11.

Tan, Alexis S. 1986. "Social Learning of Aggression from Television." pp. 41–55 in *Perspectives on Media Effects*, edited by Jennings Bryant and Dolf Zillmann. Hillsdale, NJ: Lawrence Erlbaum Associates.

Tanskanen, Antti O., Jani Erola, Johanna Kallio. 2016. "Parental Resources, Sibship Size, and Educational Performance in 20 Countries: Evidence for the Compensation Model." *Cross-Cultural Research* 50(5):452–477.

Taylor, Carl S., Richard M. Lerner, Alexander von Eye, Deborah L. Bobek, Aida B. Balsano, Elizabeth M. Dowling, and Pamela M. Anderson. 2003. "Positive Individual and Social Behavior among Gang and Nongang African American Male Adolescents." *Journal of Adolescent Research* 18(5):496–522.

Teigen, K. H., H. T. E. Normann, J. O. Bjorkheim, and S. Helland. 2000. "Who Would You Most Like to Like? Adolescents' Ideals at the Beginning and the End of the Century." *Scandinavian Journal of Educational Research* 44(1):5–26.

Tellegen, A., and G. Atkinson. 1974. "Openness to Absorbing and Self-Altering Experiences ("absorption"), a Trait Related to Hypnotic Susceptibility." *Journal of Abnormal Psychology* 83(3):268.

Terenzini, Patrick T., Leonard Springer, Ernest T. Pascarella, and Amaury Nora. 1993. "Influences Affecting the Development of Students' Critical Thinking Skills." Paper presented at the meeting of the Association for Institutional Research, New Orleans, LA.

Thomas, R. Murray. 2001. *Recent Theories of Human Development*. Thousand Oaks, CA: Sage.

Thomas, Sandra P. 1997. "Psychosocial Correlates of Womens' Self-rated Physical Health in Midlife Adulthood." pp. 257–291 in *Multiple Paths of Midlife Development*, edited by Margie E. Lachman, and Jacquelyn Boone James. Chicago, IL: University of Chicago Press.

Thompson, Martie P., and Fran H. Norris. 1992. "Crime, Social Status, and Alienation." *American Journal of Community Psychology* 20(1):97–119.

Thompson, Melissa, and Milena Petrovic. 2009. "Gendered Transitions: Within-Person Changes in Employment, Family, and Illicit Drug Use." *Journal of Research in Crime and Delinquency* 46(3):377–408.

Thornton, Patricia H., William Ocasio, and Michael Lounsbury. 2012. *The Institutional Logics Perspective: A New Approach to Culture, Structure, and Process*. Oxford, UK: Oxford University Press.

Tinsley, Brian, and Margaret Beale Spencer. 2010. "High Hope and Low Regard: The Resiliency of Adolescents' Educational Expectations While Developing in Challenging Political Contexts." *Research in Human Development* 7(3):183–201.

To, Siu-ming, Hau-lin Tam, Steven Sek-yum Ngai, and Wai-leung Sung. 2014. "Sense of Meaningfulness, Sources of Meaning, and Self-Evaluation of Economically Disadvantaged Youth in Hong Kong: Implications for Youth Development Programs." *Children and Youth Services Review* 47(3):352–361.

Toffoletti, K. 2017. "Advertising the 2015 Cricket World Cup: Representing Multicultural Female Sports Fans." *Communication & Sport*, 5(2):226–244.

Tokar, David M., Jason R. Withrow, Rosalie J. Hull, and Bonnie Moradi. 2003. "Psychological Separation, Attachment Security, Vocational Self-concept Crystallization, and Career Indecision: A Structural Equation Analysis." *Journal of Counseling Psychology* 50(1):3–19.

Tokar, David M., Mindi N. Thompson, Melissa R. Plaufcan, and Christine M. Williams. 2007. "Precursors of Learning Experiences in Social Cognitive Career Theory." *Journal of Vocational Behavior* 71:319–339.

Torfing, Jacob. 1999. *New Theories of Discourse: Laclau, Mouffe and Zizek*. Oxford, UK: Blackwell.

Toro-Morn, Maura, and Susan Sprecher. 2003. "A Cross-cultural Comparison of Mate Preferences among University Students: The United States vs. the People's Republic of China (PRC)." *Journal of Comparative Family Studies* 34(2):151–170.

Trentmann, Frank. 2007. "Citizenship and Consumption." *Journal of Consumer Culture* 7(2):147–158.

Tricarico, Giorgio. 2016. "The Individuation Process in Post-Modernity." *Psychological Perspectives* 59(4):461–472.

Tse, Thomas Kwan Choi. 2007. "Remaking Chinese Identity: Hegemonic Struggles over National Education in Post-colonial Hong Kong." *International Studies in Sociology of Education* 17(3):231–248.

Tseng, S. M. 2011. *Idol Worship, Attachment, Self-Esteem, and Loneliness: A Study among 197 Adolescents (Secondary School and University Students) in Hong Kong*. Undergraduate Thesis, City University of Hong Kong.

Tsou, Meng-Wen, and Jin-Tan Liu. 2001. "Happiness and Domain Satisfaction in Taiwan." *Journal of Happiness Studies* 2(3):269–288.

Turner, John R. 1993. "Interpersonal and Psychological Predictors of Parasocial Interaction with Different Television Performers." *Communication Quarterly* 41(4):443–453.

Turner, Jonathan H. 1986. *The Structure of Sociological Theory*, 4th ed. Belmont, CA: Wadsworth.

Turner, Sean, and Avraham Scherman. 1996. "Big Brothers' Impact on Little Brothers' Self-concepts and Behaviors." *Adolescence* 31(124):875–882.

Turner, Sherri L., Jason C. Steward, and Richard T. Lapan. 2004. "Family Factors Associated with Sixth-grade Adolescents' Math and Science Career Interests." *Career Development Quarterly* 53:41–52.

Tuval-Mashiach, R., S. Walsh, S. Harel, and S. Shulman. 2008. "Romantic Fantasies, Cross-Gender Friendships, and Romantic Experiences in Adolescence." *Journal of Adolescent Research* 23(4):471–487.

Tyler, Tom R., Robert J. Boerkmann, Heather J. Smith, and Yuen J. Huo. 1997. *Social Justice in a Diverse Society*. Boulder, CO: Westview.

Unger, Jennifer B., Louise Ann Rohrbach, Beth Howard-Pitney, Anamara Ritt-Olson, and Michele Mottapa. 2001. "Peer Influences and Susceptibility to Smoking among California Adolescents." *Substance Use & Misuse* 36(5):551–571.

Valdivia, Ibis Alvarez, Barry H. Schneider, Kenia Lorenzo Chavez, and Xinyin Chen. 2005. "Social Withdrawal and Maladjustment in a Very Group-oriented Society." *International Journal of Behavioral Development* 29(3):219–228.

Valentine, Gill. 1999. "Eating in: Home, Consumption and Identity." *Sociological Review* 47(3):491–524.

van de Ven, Niels, Marcel Zeelenberg, and Rik Pieters. 2011. "Why Envy Outperforms Admiration." *Personality & Social Psychology Bulletin* 37(6):784–795.

van de Ven, Niels. 2017. "Envy and Admiration: Emotion and Motivation Following Upward Social Comparison." *Cognition & Emotion* 31(1):193–200.

van de Werfhorst, Herman G., and Gerbert Kraaykamp. 2001. "Four Field-related Educational Resources and Their Impact on Labor, Consumption, and Sociopolitical Orientation." *Sociology of Education* 74:296–317.

van Goethem, Anne A. J., Anne van Hoof, Marcel A. G. van Aken, Quinten A. W. Raaijmakers, Jan Boom, and Bram Orobio de Castro. 2012. "The Role of Adolescents' Morality and Identity in Volunteering: Age and Gender Differences in a Process Model." *Journal of Adolescence* 35:509–520.

van Lier, Pol A. C., Frank Vitaro, Brigitte Wanner, Patricia Vuijk, and Alfons A. M. Crijnen. 2005. "Gender Differences in Developmental Links among Antisocial Behavior, Friends' Antisocial Behavior, and Peer Rejection in Childhood: Results from Two Cultures." *Child Development* 76(4):841–885.

van Zalk, Maarten Herman Walter, Margaret Kerr, Susan J. T. Branje, Hakan Stattin, and Wim H. J. Meeus. 2010. "Peer Contagion and Adolescent Depression: The Role of Failure Anticipation." *Journal of Clinical Child & Adolescent Psychology* 39(6):837–848.

Verhagen, Stijn, Frits Van Wel, Tom ter Bogt, and Belinda Hibbel. 2000. "Fast on 200 Beats per Minute: The Youth Culture of Gabbers in the Netherlands." *Youth & Society* 32(2):147–164.

Vignoli, Emmanuelle, Sandrine Croity-Belz, Valerie Chapeland, Anne de Fillipis, and Martine Garcia. 2005. "Career Exploration in Adolescents: The Role of Anxiety, Attachment, and Parenting Style." *Journal of Vocational Behavior* 67:153–168.

Vitaro, Frank, Mara Brendgen, and Brigitte Wanner. 2005. "Patterns of Affiliation with Delinquent Friends during Late Childhood and Early Adolescence: Correlates and Consequences." *Social Development* 14(1):82–108.

Vivona, Jeanine M. 2000. "Parental Attachment Styles of Late Adolescents: Qualities of Attachment Relationships and Consequences for Adjustment." *Journal of Counseling Psychology* 47(3):316–329.

Vowell, Paul R., and David C. May. 2000. "Another Look at Classic Strain Theory: Poverty Status, Perceived Blocked Opportunity, and Gang Membership as Predictors of Adolescent Violent Behavior." *Sociological Inquiry* 70(1):42–60.

Walker, Christopher O., Barbara A. Greene, and Robert A. Mansell. 2006. "Identification with Academics, Intrinsic/Extrinsic Motivation, and Self-Efficacy as Predictors of Cognitive Engagement." *Learning & Individual Differences* 16(1):1–12.

Walker, Lawrence J., and Jeremy A. Frimer. 2009. "Moral Personality Exemplified." pp. 232–255 in *Personality, Identity, and Character: Explorations in Moral Psychology*, edited by Darcin Narvaez and Daniel K. Lapsley. New York: Cambridge University Press.

Walkner, Paul, and Nicholas Finney. 1999. "Skill Development and Critical Thinking in Higher Education." *Teaching in Higher Education* 4(4):531–547.

Walstad, William B., Ken Rebeck, Richard A. MacDonald. 2010. "The Effects of Financial Education on the Financial Knowledge of High School Students." *Journal of Consumer Affairs* 44(2):336–357.

Wan, M. P. 1997. "Constructing Love Relationship with Idols." *Hong Kong Anthropologist* 10:25–31.

Wang, Alvin Y. 1994. "Pride and Prejudice in High School Gang Members." *Adolescence* 29(114):279–291.

Wang, Chia-chen, Chin-ta Chen, Shu-chen Yang, Cheng-kiang Farn. 2009. "Pirate or Buy? The Moderating Effect of Idolatry." *Journal of Business Ethics* 90(1):81–93.

Wang, Danyu. 2004. "Ritualistic Coresidence and the Weakening of Filial Practice in Rural China." pp. 16–33 in *Filial Piety: Practice and Discourses in Contemporary East Asia*, edited by Charlotte Ikels. Stanford, CA: Stanford University Press.

Wang, Peigang, and Tyler J. VanderWeele. 2011. "Empirical Research on Factors Related to the Subjective Well-being of Chinese Urban Residents." *Social Indicators Research* 101:447–459.

Wang, Qi, Stacey N. Doan, and Qinfang Song. 2010. "Talking about Internet States in Mother-Child Reminiscing Influences Children's Self-representations: A Cross-cultural Study." *Cognitive Development* 25:380–393.

Wang, Zheng. 2008. "National Humiliation, History Education, and the Politics of Historical Memory: Patriotic Education Campaign in China." *International Studies Quarterly* 52:783–806.

Wang, Zhengping, and Minyan Zhu. 1996. *Wisdom of Goodness: Insight into Traditional Moral Theories of China*. Shanghai, China: Fudan University.

Ward, Mary J., Shelley S. Lee, and H. Jonathan Polan. 2006. "Attachment and Psychopathology in a Community Sample." *Attachment & Human Development* 8(4):327–340.

Warr, Mark. 2005. "Making Delinquent Friends: Adult Supervision and Children's Affiliations." *Criminology* 43(1):77–105.

Waterman, A. S., and S. L. Archer. 1993. "Identity Status during the Adult Years: Scoring Criteria." pp. 241–279 in *Ego Identity: A Handbook for Psychosocial Research*, edited by J. E. Marcia, A. S. Waterman, D. R. Matterson, S. L. Archer, and J. L. Orlofsky. New York: Springer-Verlag.

Waterman, A. S., and C. K. Waterman. 1972. "Relationship between Freshman Ego Identity Status and Subsequent Academic Behavior: A Test of the Predictive Validity of Marcia's Categorization System for Identity Status." *Developmental Psychology* 6(1):179.

Watson, Cary M., Teri Quatman, and Erik Edler. 2002. "Career Aspirations of Adolescent Girls: Effects of Achievement Level, Grade, and Single-sex School Environment." *Sex Roles* 46(9/10):323–335.

Watt, Helen M. G., Colin Carmichael, and Rosemary Callingham. 2017. "Students' Engagement Profiles in Mathematics According to Learning Environment Dimensions: Developing an Evidence Base for Best Practice in Mathematics Education." *School Psychology International* 38(2):166–183.

Wearden, A., I. Peters, K. Berry, C. Barrowdough, and T. Liversidge. 2008. "Adult Attachment, Parenting Experiences, and Core Beliefs about Self and Others." *Personality and Individual Differences* 44:1246–1257. doi:10.1016/j.paid.2007.11.019

Weems, Carl F., Steven L. Berman, Wendy K. Silverman, and Eileen T. Rodriguez. 2002. "The Relation between Anxiety Sensitivity and Attachment Style in Adolescence and Early Adulthood." *Journal of Psychopathology & Behavioral Assessment* 24(3):159–168.

Weiss, R. S. 1973. Loneliness: The Experience of Emotional and Social Isolation.

Wen, Nainan, and Di Cui. 2014. "Effects of Celebrity Involvement on Young People's Political and Civic Engagement." *Chinese Journal of Communication*. 7(4):409–428.

Wexler, Harry K., Gregory P. Falkin, and Douglas S. Lipton. 1990. "Outcome Evaluation of a Prison Therapeutic Community for Substance Abuse Treatment." *Criminal Justice and Behavior* 17(1):71–92.

White, Mark H., II, and Ludwin E. Molina. 2016. "Infrahumanizing Praise: Athletic Admiration Decreases Perceptions of Agency and Support for College Athletes' Rights." *Social Psychology* 47(4):187–200.

White, Steven H., and Joseph H. O'Brien. 1999. "What Is a Hero? An Exploratory Study of Students' Conceptions of Heroes." *Journal of Moral Education* 28(1):81–95.

Whyte, Martin King, and Maocan Gao. 2009. "How Angry Are Chinese Citizens about Current Inequalities? Evidence from a National Survey." *Social Transformations in Chinese Societies* 5:17–54.

Wiesner, Margit, and Hyoun K. Kim. 2006. "Co-occurring Delinquency and Depressive Symptoms of Adolescent Boys and Girls: A Dual Trajectory Modeling Approach." *Developmental Psychology* 42(6):1220–1235.

Wilder, David H., Huhg F. McKeegan, and Robert M. Midkiffe, Jr. 2000. "A Factor-analytic Reinterpretation of the Clark-Trow Educational Philosophies." *Journal of College Student Development* 41(5):513–528.

Wilkinson, Derek. 2008. "Individual and Community Factors Affecting Psychological Sense of Community, Attraction and Neighboring in Rural Communities." *Canadian Review of Sociology* 45(3):305–329.

Wilkinson, R. B. 2004. "The Role of Parental and Peer Attachment in the Psychological Health and Self-esteem of Adolescents." *Journal of Youth and Adolescence* 33(6):479–493.

Wilkinson, Ross B. 2010. "Best Friend Attachment versus Peer Attachment in the Prediction of Adolescent Psychological Adjustment." *Journal of Adolescence* 33(5):709–717.

Willis, S. E. 1972. "Falling in Love with Celebrities." *Sexual Behavior* 2:2–8.

Wilson, Glenn D. 1973. *The Psychology of Conservatism*. London: Academic Press.

Wilson, John. 2000. "Volunteering." *Annual Review of Sociology* 26:215–240.

Winnicott, D. W. 1965. *The Maturational Process and the Facilitating Environment*. New York: International Universities Press.

Winters, Ken C., Randy D. Stinchfield, and Leigh G. Kim. 1995. "Monitoring Adolescent Gambling in Minnesota." *Journal of Gambling Studies* 11(2):165–183.

Wires, John W., Ralph Barocas, and Albert R. Hollenbeck. 1994. "Determinants of Adolescent Identity Development: A Cross-sequential Study of Boarding School Boys." *Adolescence* 29(114):361–378.

Wiseman, H., O. Mayseless, and R. Sharabany. 2006. "Why Are They Lonely? Perceived Quality of Early Relationships with Parents, Attachment, Personality Predispositions and Loneliness in First-year University Students." *Personality and Individual Differences* 40(2):237–248.

Wong, S. W., and K. Ma. 1997. A Survey on the Patterns of Canto-Pop Appreciation in Hong Kong. Department of Applied Social Studies, City University of Hong Kong.

Woodward, Lianne J., and David M. Fergusson. 1999. "Childhood Peer Relationship Problems and Psychosocial Adjustment in Late Adolescence." *Journal of Abnormal Child Psychology* 27(1):87–124.

Wouters, Sofie, Hilde Colpin, Jan Van Damme, Steven De Laet, and Karine Verschueren. 2013. "Early Adolescents' Academic Self-concept Formation: Do Classmates or Friends Matter Most?" *Learning & Individual Differences* 27:193–200.

Wright, Darlene R., and Kevin M. Fitzpatrick. 2006. "Social Capital and Adolescent Violent Behavior: Correlates of Fighting and Weapon Use among Secondary School Students." *Social Forces* 84(3):1435–1453.

Wu, C. H. 2009. "The Relationship between Attachment Style and Self-concept Clarity: The Mediation Effect of Self-esteem." *Personality and Individual Differences* 47(1):42–46.

Wu, D. 2003. *Moral Education Curriculum and Education*. Hangzhou, China: Jiejiang.

Wu, Joseph, and Dennis S. W. Wong. 2013. "Psychosocial Corelates of Friendship in School." pp. 159–168 in *Friendships: Cultural Variations, Developmental Issues and Impact on Health*, edited by Sarah Kaufman and Viktor Meyer. New York: Nova.

Wu, Michael Shengtao, Xiaodan Yan, Chan Zhou, Yiwen Chen, Juan Li, Zhuohong Zhu, Xiangqin Shen, and Buxin Han. 2010. "General Belief in a Just World and Resilience: Evidence from a Collectivistic Culture." *European Journal of Personality* 25(6):431–442.

Wu, Tsu-Yin, Nola Pender, and Samar Noureddine. 2003. "Gender Differences in the Psychosocial and Cognitive Correlates of Physical Activity among Taiwanese Adolescents: A Structural Equation Modeling Approach." *International Journal of Behavioral Medicine* 10(2):93–105.

Wyman, Peter A. 2003. "Emerging Perspectives on Context Specificity of Children's Adaptation and Resilience: Evidence from a Decade of Research with Urban Children in Adversity." pp. 293–317 in *Resilience and Vulnerability: Adaptation in the Context of Childhood Adversities*, edited by Saniya S. Luthar. Cambridge, UK: Cambridge University Press.

Xue, Xiao-Yang. 1997. "Idol Education: New Concepts in Educational Theories (in Chinese)." *Educational Commentary (in Chinese), Fu Zhou* 1:22–25.

Yeh, Kuang-Hui, and Yung-Jui Yang. 2006. "Construct Validation of Individuating and Relating Autonomy Orientations in Culturally Chinese Adolescents." *Asian Journal of Social Psychology* 9(2):148–160.

Yi, Chin-Chun, Chin-Fen Chang, and Ying-Hwa Chang. 2004. "The Intergenerational Transmission of Family Values: A Comparison between Teenagers and Parents in Taiwan." *Journal of Comparative Family Studies* 35(4):523–545.

Yon, Kyu Jin, Ju-ri Joeng, and Michael Goh. 2012. "A Longitudinal Study of Career Maturity of Korean Adolescents: The Effects of Personal and Contextual Factors." *Asia Pacific Education Review* 13(4):727–739.

Youniss, James, and Miranda Yates. 1997. *Community Service and Social Responsibility in Youth*. Chicago, IL: University of Chicago Press.

Youniss, James, and Miranda Yates. 1999. "Youth Service and Moral-civic Identity: A Case for Everyday Morality." *Educational Psychology Review* 11(4):361–376.

Yue, X. D. 1999. "Comparing Idol Worship and Model Emulation in Youth and Adolescence." *Journal of Youth Studies* 4(2):91–98.

Yue, X. D., and C. K. Cheung. 2000a. "Idol Worshipping and Model Learning among Chinese Young People: A Comparative Study among Students in Hong Kong, Guangzhou and Changsha." *Journal of Youth Studies (Hong Kong)* 3:133–145.

Yue, X. D., and C. K. Cheung. 2000b. "Selection of Favourite Idols and Models among Chinese Young People: A Comparative Study in Hong Kong and Nanjing." *International Journal of Behavioral Development* 24:91–98.

Yue, X. D., and C. K. Cheung. 2002. "Worshiping Star Idols and Luminary Idols: Reflections of 1998–2001 Studies in Hong Kong and Mainland China." *Journal of Youth Studies (Hong Kong)* 5:179–191.

Yue, X. D., C. K. Cheung, and S. W. Wong. 2003. "Impacts of Gender and Age on Adolescent Idol Worship: A Study in Hong Kong and Mainland China." *Educational Research Journal* 18:97–111.

Yue, X. D., C. K. Cheung, and D. S. W. Wong. 2010. "From Glamour-Oriented Idolatry to Achievement-Oriented Idolatry: A Framing Experiment among Adolescents in Hong Kong and Shenzhen." *Asian Journal of Social Psychology* 13(1):1–8.

Yue, X. D., and X. Liang. 2009. "Series Discussion of Adolescent Idolatery Four: On the Classification of Adolescent Idolatry." *Youth Studies* 3(8): 53–59.

Yue, X. D., S. W. Wong, and C. K. "Cheung. 2000. Survey and Analysis of Differences in Idolatry between Secondary School Students in Hong Kong and Mainland." *Hong Kong Journal of Social Work* 34:57–72.

Yurchisin, Jennifer, Yoo Jin Kwon, and Sara B. Marcketti. 2009. "Consumers of Charity Bracelets: Cause-supporters or Fashion-followers?" *Journal of Fashion Marketing & Management* 13(3):448–457.

Zeidner, Moshe, Gerald Matthews, and Richard D. Roberts. 2009. *What We Know about Emotional Intelligence: How It Affects Learning, Work, Relationships, and Our Mental Health.* Cambridge, MA: MIT.

Zemba, Yuriko, and Maia J. Young. 2012. "Assigning Credit to Organizational Leaders: How Japanese and Americans Differ." *Journal of Cross-cultural Psychology* 43(6):899–914.

Zeng, Zhen, and Yu Xie. 2008. "A Preference-Opportunity-Choice Framework with Applications to Intergroup Friendship." *American Journal of Sociology* 114(3):615–648.

Zhan, Wangsheng, and Wujie Ning. 2004. "The Moral Education Curriculum for Junior High Schools in 21st Century China." *Journal of Moral Education* 33(4):511–532.

Zhang, Jie, and Darwin L. Thomas. 1994. "Modernization Theory Revisited: A Cross-cultural Study of Adolescent Conformity to Significant Others in Mainland China, Taiwan, and the USA." *Adolescence* 29:885–903.

Zhang, Lifang. 2008. "Revisiting the Big Six and the Big Five among Hong Kong University Students." *Educational Psychology* 28(1):1–14.

Zhang, Shixin. 2003. *Moral Education and Four Great Realms: Comparative Study of Sects of China's Ancient Moral Education.* Hangzhou, China: Zhejiang Educational.

Zhou, Qing, Nancy Eisenberg, Yun Wang, and Mark Reiser. 2004. "Chinese Children's Effortful Control and Disposition Anger/Frustration, Relations to Parenting Styles and Children's Social Functioning." *Developmental Psychology* 40(3):352–366.

Zhu, Xiaoman, 2006. "Moral Education and Values Education in Curriculum Reform in China." *Frontier of Education in China* 2:191–200.

Zimmer-Gembeck, Melanie J., Nicole Hughes, Marguerite Kelly, and Jennifer Connolly. 2012. "Intimacy, Identity and Status: Measuring Dating Goals in Late Adolescence and Emerging Adulthood." *Motivation & Emotion* 36(3):311–322.

Zukin, Sharon. 1998. "Urban Lifestyles: Diversity and Standardisation in Spaces of Consumption." *Urban Studies* 35(5–6):825–839.

Zupancic, Maja, Luka Komidar, and Melita Puklek Levpuscek. 2014. "Individuation in Slovene Emerging Adults: Its Associations with Demographics, Transitional Markers, Achieved Criteria for Adulthood, and Life Satisfaction." *Journal of Adolescence* 37(8):1421–1433.

Zysberg, Leehu. 2012. "Loneliness and Emotional Intelligence." *Journal of Psychology* 146(1–2):37–46.

Index